UNIT MEDICAL RECORDS

UNIT MEDICAL RECORDS

In Hospital and Clinic

By DOROTHY L. KURTZ

New York : Morningside Heights
COLUMBIA UNIVERSITY PRESS

Copyright 1943, Columbia University Press, New York

First printing 1943
Second printing 1950

Published in Great Britain, Canada, and India
by Geoffrey Cumberlege, Oxford University Press,
London, Toronto, and Bombay

Manufactured in the United States of America

CONTENTS

I. **DEFINITION AND HISTORY** — 1
History of Medical Records; Summary

II. **CONTENT AND FORM** — 11
Front Unit or Index Sheet; Chronological Record; Series of Examinations and Treatments; Supplementary Progress Notes; Summary Sheets; Format; Summary

III. **MAINTENANCE** — 34
Identifying the Case; Period of Hospitalization; Assistance for the Doctor; Maintaining the Record Standard; Summary

IV. **FILING AND TRANSPORTATION** — 45
Filing Scheme; Space and Housing; Requisition-filler System; Transportation of Records; Filing Schedule; Summary

V. **INDEXING** — 61
Name Index; Diagnostic and Treatment Index; The Standard Nomenclature as a Basis for Indexing; Secondary Indexes; Summary

VI. **RIGHTS, RESPONSIBILITIES, AND SAFEGUARDS** — 79
Functions of the Record; Position of the Parties Concerned; Safeguards within the Institution; Dealing with Outsiders; Subpoenaed Records; Summary

VII. **SOURCE OF STUDY MATERIAL** — 90
Collecting Research Data; Tabulating the Material; Other Types of Studies; Summary

INDEX — 103

FIGURES

1.	Front Unit Sheet	13
2.	Graphic or Temperature Chart	23
3.	Admission and Discharge Sheet	28
4.	Record Bag	57
5.	Name Index Card	62
6.	Diagnostic Index Card	67
7.	Section of Diagnostic Index	76
8.	Sample Statistical Summary Form	93–94

NOTE TO THE SECOND PRINTING

Since the record system described here remains basically the same, a revised edition of this book has been unnecessary. However, two important developments that have taken place since the book was first published in 1943 have been included in this reprinting by revision of pages 49–53. Reverse numerical filing offers many advantages over the conventional system of filing hospital records. Likewise the development of shelving especially adapted to medical records promises both to save space and to promote convenience. Both discussions contribute additional value to the book.

D. L. K.

The Presbyterian Hospital
in the City of New York
January 3, 1950

I. DEFINITION AND HISTORY

IN ORDER TO UNDERSTAND why the unit medical record deserves consideration apart from medical records in general, we need to appreciate just what it is. Were it merely an improved filing scheme, it would surely not warrant this attention. Its significance is much more deeply rooted. It is, in fact, the practical expression of a fundamental medical concept, that the individual—not some part of him or some episode in his history, but the whole individual—is the *unit* of medical practice and study. There is nothing new in this idea. The question never arose until the rapid growth of specialized medicine and of hospitalization destroyed the unity and the continuity of the family doctor's approach. As this loss was felt the medical profession set to work to develop some means of correlating the findings on a given patient, made at different times and by different special services—at least within each institution. The result is the unit medical record. That it was developed by doctors themselves to fill a definite need and has since come to be so widely accepted by them as the ideal form of hospital record is the best evidence of its soundness. This recognition has come about, too, on its own merits and without any organized fanfare.

Along with this unquestioning acceptance of the unit

DEFINITION AND HISTORY

medical record, however, there is a good deal of haziness about its practical possibilities and problems. To attempt to install this type of record in a hospital without understanding the difficulties as well as the advantages which are peculiar to it is very apt to lead to discouragement. Indeed, most criticism has arisen when the unit system has been adopted on a wave of enthusiasm, but under physical arrangements which rendered its operation all but impossible. Nothing is clearer than that each institution must adapt its record system carefully to fit its own peculiar organization, type of patient, type of staff, and physical layout and equipment. Nevertheless, certain principles capable of general application have emerged during the twenty-five years since the unit record was first put into effect in the Presbyterian Hospital in New York. We shall attempt, then, to winnow from this experience those essentials of the unit record which characterize it under any circumstances.

HISTORY OF MEDICAL RECORDS

We will appreciate many things in our study of the unit record much better, if we pause first to take a quick glance at the history of medical records in general. While treatises on disease by the Egyptians are believed by some to date as far back as 4500 B.C., the first detailed case reports of which we know are those of Hippocrates (born about 460 B.C.). He was the first to proclaim that disease arises from natural causes, not from acts of the gods. It is no coincidence that the first man to approach medicine as a science was also the first to leave careful records. His genius consisted in rejecting current superstition and in basing his deductions

DEFINITION AND HISTORY

upon his own careful observations. These observations, moreover, he preserved from the distortions of memory by prompt recording. Except for laboratory and instrumental reports, his physical examinations and progress notes are ridiculously like those of today. From his day to this, wherever the care of the sick has been undertaken on a scientific level rather than that of witchcraft or even that of charity alone, some form of patient's record has resulted.

As long as the general practitioner was able to attend to all or most of his patients' needs, there was no problem of records. He kept what he felt necessary, and that was all there was to it. As medical science gathered momentum, however, one man could no longer master the entire field and specialization was inevitable. For the same reason, more and more patients were sent to hospitals to receive the more elaborate treatments impossible at home. Quite naturally, at first there was no thought of hospital records apart from registration. Medical records were still considered the responsibility of each doctor. More than a trace of this attitude still persists in regard to private patients' records. However, just as soon as the care of patients came to be shared by attending doctor, intern, and specialist, the value of such experience for teaching and study was recognized. Records of unusual cases were being kept at the beginning of the nineteenth century by the Pennsylvania Hospital in Philadelphia and by the New York Hospital. By the latter part of the century, it had become approved practice to keep patients' records routinely. The responsibility had also shifted from the individual doctor to the hospital, so that the whole staff might share in their joint experience.

Now the problem became one of organizing this accumulating material so that it could be used. Hospital records of the late 1800's and early 1900's bear evidence of this trial-and-error period. To begin with, the records were merely stored in bundles, or, in more particular institutions, bound chronologically in great heavy volumes. Soon name indexes were included in each volume, and before long special index volumes were set up for names, diagnoses, and operations. In order to make research on certain diseases easier, Bellevue Hospital evolved the scheme of binding together all records with the same diagnosis. Card files for both name and diagnostic indexes appeared next, reflecting the rapid replacement in the business world of ledgers by modern card and vertical filing. The Massachusetts General Hospital took an important step in 1897 when it employed a competent librarian who was to include in her duties the care and indexing of the medical records. This lead was not followed generally for a good many years, however. It was rare indeed for a hospital of this period to employ anyone specifically to care for its records. What was achieved was done by interested members of the professional staff who gave their own time and borrowed any help they could from whatever clerical staff the hospital possessed.

One specific movement effecting the organization of medical records came very much to the fore just after the turn of the twentieth century. This was the matter of a uniform diagnostic nomenclature, the use of which by all members of a hospital staff greatly simplifies the indexing of case records. Several good ones were brought out independently, those by Massachusetts General and Bellevue Hospitals being the best known. Just how much they were inspired by the International Cause of Death List, which was ac-

DEFINITION AND HISTORY

cepted in this country about the same time, is hard to say. Both were shortly revised to conform to it, however. The wide adoption of these nomenclatures by other hospitals bespeaks the need they filled.

Up to this point the advances had all been in the matter of preserving and indexing medical records. It was still a formidable task to assemble any number of cases of a given condition or even to examine the progress of a single patient. To do either meant handling numbers of heavy volumes. To find out what was being done for a patient in the out-patient department multiplied the difficulties. There it was the common practice for each service to keep its own separate record file, and all of these, of course, were apart from the hospital records. Thus to collect the data on a patient with a history of repeated admissions and varied clinic care was exceedingly laborious. To attempt it for many cases was out of the question. Perhaps this lack of continuity was most felt by the surgeons, who had no satisfactory way of determining the final result of their operations. At any rate, it was obvious that neither the members of a hospital's staff nor its patients were getting anywhere near the benefits which should be derived from this association of trained professional minds. Finally in 1916 the Presbyterian Hospital in New York began the operation of its unit record system. That this was actually the first is uncertain, but the care with which it was worked out and the wide interest it aroused establish its significance. At last a doctor could ask for a group of cases by name or by diagnosis and receive them, each in a convenient folder. Not only were notes on all the admissions of a patient bound together, but, if he had ever attended clinic, these notes appeared chronologically among the hospital ones. Included also were follow-up notes at varying intervals. In fact, a careful follow-up scheme was tied in with the unit record system from the beginning. So many inquiries regarding this system were received that an illustrated reprint of reports on it was issued and widely distributed both in this country and abroad.

About the same time, but from an entirely different source, a movement developed which was to bring home to the most remote hospitals in the country the importance of keeping their records complete and available. In 1913 the American College of Surgeons was organized, with the purpose of establishing a standard for surgical work. Each candidate for a fellowship was required to submit a number of case records of patients upon whom he had operated, as evidence of his ability and judgment. It immediately appeared, however, that few hospitals could furnish records of any value for this purpose. In fact, it became evident that the standard of surgery could not be greatly raised without attention to the conditions under which it was performed, in other words, to those prevailing in the hospitals. Accordingly in 1918 this organization incorporated practices which had developed independently in the best hospitals into their "Minimum Standard Requirements." These called for a fully qualified professional staff to be organized and to hold meetings at least monthly for the purpose of analyzing their clinical experience. Since the basis of this analysis was of necessity the medical record, just what this should include was indicated. The proper diagnostic and therapeutic facilities were also outlined. Later recommendations set forth types of indexes considered essential. In accord with this standard, hospitals are rated annually by the American College of Surgeons. The American Medical Association and the American Hospital Association have also been active in this campaign of improvement, although these have never been quite so closely concerned with the records. The real contribution of all these organizations toward improving medical records has not been in developing a system, but in *promoting* approved methods among the more backward institutions.

Their efforts they found seriously hampered by the lack of suitable personnel in the record field. Therefore in 1928 the American College of Surgeons sponsored the organization of what is now the American Association of Medical Record Librarians. Working at first under the close tutelage of the parent organization, this group has gradually taken over the functions of advancing and standardizing the quality of medical records. Local discussion groups were one of the earliest and most effective means of spreading knowledge among those actually engaged in record work. To establish a standard for such people, the association very soon set up a registry for record librarians. Acceptance is based upon special education or experience in record work and the passing of a written examination. Likewise the American Association established and supervise closely a number of training schools. Requirements are high, and the student receives at least nine months' practical training, supplemented by lectures in related subjects.

In none of the activities of these organizations has the unit record been especially stressed. In fact, in early discussions its advantages were often disputed, and several important hospitals were slow in adopting it. Nevertheless,

8 DEFINITION AND HISTORY

out of all the attention focused upon medical records in general, it has emerged the accepted type. Those hospitals using other systems do so now not from conviction but because of practical difficulties. Obviously no matter how satisfactory the record itself may be, it is useless unless it can be promptly produced wherever it is required. Proper filing space and location are the root of the problem. So serious are these factors that not even in the hospital where the unit system originated could it be carried to its logical conclusion until that hospital and its associate institutions moved into their new buildings at the Columbia-Presbyterian Medical Center. Then, thirteen years after individual records had been combined, it became possible to unify the entire out-patient and hospital files into a single numerical system. At the same time a master name index was formed from the separate indexes, and likewise a master diagnostic index. As other hospitals joined, their records, too, were merged into this central filing system. Improvements in handling the records were also inaugurated at this time in order to meet the greatly increased problems of circulation. Thus was achieved not only a unit record, but a unified record system.

One other influence has begun to effect medical records and probably will become increasingly important. This is the interest which public health agencies of all types have in hospital records as a source of statistical material. Mortality data have long been available through the required registration of deaths, but general morbidity data are most difficult to obtain. The idea of tapping hospital records for this purpose lay behind the establishment of the *Standard Classified Nomenclature of Disease*. It was felt that a com-

DEFINITION AND HISTORY

mon language of disease should be the first step in this direction. Accordingly in 1928 the National Conference on Nomenclature of Disease was formed, with the sole purpose of establishing a representative nomenclature. Practically all of the national medical associations were given an opportunity to participate in its construction. After two editions were published the conference dissolved in 1937, and a permanent organization was arranged under the American Medical Association. Whatever its faults, the Standard Nomenclature did achieve two things of great value. It did represent the opinion of specialist groups and of various sections of the country instead of just a single institution. Also, a permanent clearing house was set up to consider questions and suggestions from all its users and to handle periodic revisions.

SUMMARY

Medical records are not imposed upon the medical profession from without, but are the natural accompaniment of the scientific approach. Every important development in the records themselves has come from individual hospital staffs which were striving to meet a practical need. They urged the hospitals to preserve patients' records in the first place, suggested indexing them, and contributed the first nomenclatures to make indexing more accurate. They, too, evolved the unit record to correlate for treatment and study the scattered material on a single patient. The system of keeping records has been improved by nonprofessional individuals responsible for this phase of the work, and promoting all these advances has been the function of the national organizations interested in this field. The interest of public health groups in medical records as a source of morbidity statistics is just beginning to make itself felt, but it already accounts for the development of a representative nomenclature of disease.

II. CONTENT AND FORM

MERELY to collect in a single folder all the data on one patient does not accomplish the purpose of a unit record. This material must be so arranged and presented that one can find any particular kind of note among all the others and do it quickly. Also the general outline of the case should be apparent at once without the necessity of searching. This is no problem in a record dealing with a single admission, but in one covering any number of hospital admissions, plus attendance in various out-patient services, the matter is anything but simple. Those who developed the original unit record gave very careful consideration to this problem of organizing the material in it, and subsequent experience has indicated no fundamental change in their plan.

Since their idea in developing the unit record was to emphasize the progress of the entire patient, they made their basic arrangement chronological. The common plan of grouping together all notes of each type, such as all operations, all laboratory reports, and so forth, obviously tends to departmentalize the material and to destroy its unity, however convenient it may be to follow progress in a given line. Certain notes warrant such separation for very good reasons, but they are made the exception rather than the rule, as we shall see.

CONTENT AND FORM

It should be understood that the arrangement of which we speak refers to the final bound record. While a patient is in the hospital, the arrangement of his current admission sheets concerns only those who are working on them.

FRONT UNIT OR INDEX SHEET

This, the first sheet of the record, is invaluable in presenting at a glance the outstanding facts of the whole case. Headed simply by the patient's name and age, it is divided into two columns. In the left-hand column is typed the service and dates of admission and discharge for each period of hospitalization, together with the result. Opposite this, in the right-hand column, appear the final diagnoses and any operations performed. Also in the left column may be recorded each clinic service attended, with the date of the first visit. Whenever diagnoses are made in the clinic they also may be entered in the right column, with the dates on which they are made. This exact form for the sheet is not essential, but it can readily be seen how necessary some such outline is, in view of the variety and quantity of material in some of these records.

CHRONOLOGICAL RECORD

The chronological record begins immediately after the "front unit sheet." It proceeds from the first contact with the patient to the last, through both clinic and hospital care. It is the basic record, and as such contains a great variety of material. Probably the doctors' progress notes in both out- and in-patient departments are the main component. They are freely interlarded, however, with all kinds of special examinations, ranging from thorough work-ups to

BABIES HOSPITAL INSTITUTE OF OPHTHALMOLOGY NEUROLOGICAL INSTITUTE PRESBYTERIAN HOSPITAL SLOANE HOSPITAL FOR WOMEN VANDERBILT CLINIC		FRONT UNIT SHEET		ASSOCIATED WITH NEW YORK STATE PSYCHIATRIC INSTITUTE COLUMBIA UNIVERSITY COLLEGE OF PHYSICIANS & SURGEONS COLUMBIA UNIVERSITY SCHOOL OF DENTAL & ORAL SURGERY

Name: John Doe   Age: 44   Unit No. 598067

SERVICE	DATE	DIAGNOSES AND OPERATIONS	
SURGICAL DIAGNOSTIC	JUL 20 1942	OPD SURG DIAG: 7/21/42	Peritoneal adhesions following operation
FRACTURE	AUG 2 2 1942	OPD FRACTURE: 8/22/42	Simple fracture of shaft of humerus
ADMISSION TO SURGERY	10/29/42 - 12/3/42	HOSP DIAG:	Chronic colitis Peritoneal adhesions following operation
		OPERATION:	Exploratory laparotomy Division of peritoneal adhesions

Figure 1
FRONT UNIT SHEET

simple laboratory reports, with individual treatment reports, including operation records, with brief social notes with pertinent correspondence and with authorizations. Such an intermixing is not nearly as confusing as it might seem, for each of these various insertions has a distinctive form which renders it easy to find. At the same time, they all lend meaning to the doctors' notes among which they appear.

The various forms composing the chronological record, which we are about to describe, have evolved to fit certain situations. They are not in any sense offered as the final word, but rather as suggestions which have been found workable in this type of record.

Application data quite naturally begin the record. The first essential is a thorough identification. This is often more difficult than the uninitiated would believe. Probably the surest and simplest way to distinguish people with the same name is to obtain as a matter of routine the first name of the father and mother. Beside the address, whatever items may be needed to complete the picture and form the basis of statistical studies, such as age, sex, race, birthplace, marital state, and occupation should also be included. In addition, the hospital administration may save time and even money by asking certain other questions as a matter of routine at this point. Inquiring where the patient was previously treated may bring to light an old record or speed the process of securing past data from outside sources. The recording on each case of any accident or hospital insurance carried and the name and address of the employer in cases of injury assures collection on many compensation and insurance cases which otherwise might slip through unnoticed. If the clinic is trying to avoid competition with local doctors, a rough assessment of the patient's financial status may be needed. Finally a place is required for the admission diagnosis, or at least for the service to which the patient is assigned by the examining doctor.

All this varied data may conveniently be combined on one side of a record sheet. If the patient is accepted, this sheet can begin the record with the first professional notes on the back. If he is referred elsewhere after a brief treatment, as in some accident cases, it alone may be filed, thus preserving altogether and in very small space all that was learned about him. In a record which is to continue for years much of this data will become out of date and will need revision. The natural time to do this is on the occasion of each hospital admission. It is usually easier to fill out a compete new form at that time, which may be placed in the record with other notes for that admission. Changes of address, which are apt to occur more frequently, may simply be made on the front cover. Careful attention should be given to the wording of the questions or headings. It is amazingly difficult to formulate in a few words a query or a title which is entirely free from ambiguity. The feeling against including financial data on the medical record is simply outweighed by its convenience under some circumstances, as in a clinic where over-rate patients are ineligible for much of the care. There is less objection, too, if outsiders are not allowed to examine the records.

An initial examination covering pertinent history and physical findings is the logical starting point for any course of treatments or special investigations. Such an examination not only begins the doctors' notes for the entire record, but it is repeated from different angles every time the patient is admitted to the hospital, enters a new service in the clinic, or comes under the observation of a consultant. The outline for a thorough investigation of this type has been standardized by the national associations in the following logical order.

Complaint, as given by the patient himself, indicates the first line of inquiry.

Family history aims to bring out any hereditary tendencies with a possible bearing on the present condition.

Personal history has the same purpose with regard to the patient's own background. It is necessary to know if in his occupation or other environment he has been subject to infection, poison, or stress of any kind. What are his habits regarding sleep, exercise, eating, and stimulants? In his past life what has he experienced with respect to acute infectious diseases, allergic phenomena, injuries, respiratory, cardiac, gastrointestinal, genitourinary, and neuromuscular symptoms?

Present illness consists primarily of the patient's account of his symptoms. The doctor supplements this with pertinent questions about pain, changes in weight or bodily functions, and so forth. Here, too, it is helpful to note any treatment elsewhere for this condition, so that an abstract may be requested, if it is warranted.

Physical examination carries the inquiry into its objective phase. Some form of anatomical outline is usually followed. Under each heading the doctor notes his observations, both positive and negative. This is either a bedside or an out-patient examination, however, so that laboratory and elaborate instrumental findings have no place in it.

The provisional diagnosis is the opinion of the doctor, based solely upon the foregoing examination. It is in no way conclusive, but points the way to further study and treatment.

One difficulty recurs so often in using a long outline like this that it is worth mentioning. It is very easy so to abbreviate statements that it is not clear whether a given condition was looked for and not found or simply not looked for. To avoid this confusion, when no observation was made, it is better to omit the heading entirely or to state definitely, "not examined."

While the main headings of the initial examination have been standardized, it is obvious that circumstances would greatly affect the detail. In the case of a readmission or an admission direct from the clinic, the unit record makes it possible to abbreviate considerably, provided that the interval is adequately covered. The thoroughness of a diagnostic work-up would also be absurd in tonsillectomy or accident cases. Because there is so much variation, even among individual cases, printed forms have not proved very satisfactory. An exception may be made in cases which tend to be very uniform, as in obstetrics. Also, as in the case of neurological examinations, where the detail is extremely fine and lengthy, a printed form may be found sufficiently convenient to overcome the objection of rigidity. On the whole, however, better notes seem to result when a memorized outline is followed, with suitable adaptations for each service. A special form is unnecessary, since the written headings stand out sufficiently to distinguish this part of the record.

Progress notes form a running record of observations, conclusions, and recommendations by any doctor attending the patient. Aside from date and signature, there are no requirements as to form. In reality the state of the case dictates the frequency of the progress notes, but it has sometimes been found wise to require a note from the man in charge every few days while the patient is in the hospital to afford proof that the patient's treatment has been adequately supervised. These notes, like the initial examination, require no special sheet or printed heading. They constitute the body of the record, and everything else is distinguished from them in one way or another.

Special examination and treatment records may be handled in either of two ways, according to whether they are essentially valuable in a series or as single reports. The former condition we will consider a little later, but individual reports concern us here because they are entered in the chronological record just as they occur.

Laboratory reports, including all the various chemical and biological analyses of specimens and instrumental examinations performed by technicians, such as basal metabolism tests and even photographs, are numerically important. They are also brief, constituting merely the technicians' answers to the doctors' implied questions. They do not contain any expression of opinion. The important thing is to have them accurately recorded and as easy to find as possible. While writing them in red ink among the progress notes satisfies the latter requirement, the extra copying offers an opportunity for error. By having them written in the laboratories directly upon small stickers, it is possible for inexperienced clerks to attach them to the record according to date with great speed and but trifling danger of error. This factor of speed is most important in the out-patient work, where the quantity of such tests has been increasing by leaps and bounds. While these stickers are none too neat in appearance, an incidental advantage is that they stand out so clearly in a page of written notes. The inclusion of photographs presents a special problem, and envelopes, the size of record sheets, offer one solution.

Specialists' examinations and treatments include X-ray, operation and anesthesia reports, biopsy and autopsy reports, and consultations. In this case the value lies chiefly in the opinion or observations of a specialist. Usually these follow a definite logical form, proceeding from an examination through carefully weighed conclusions or description of procedures, as the case may be. Because of their length and importance they are usually made upon specially headed sheets which serve to distinguish them. These sheets are inserted among the progress notes as close as possible to the proper date, somewhat like illustrations in a book.

An autopsy report thus always comes at the end of the record. It is the most elaborate of all the special examinations. It begins with a complete résumé of the patient's history and treatment, continues with a gross examination of every organ and tissue, then with a microscopic examination of the same and any chemical or bacteriological tests suggested by the pathology of the case. The pathologist then summarizes the processes causing death and all structural changes discovered. He concludes with a complete list of diagnoses covering clinical as well as anatomical abnormalities. So much does such a study add to the value of the record that it should always be included in its entirety, not merely the resulting diagnoses.

Very informal consultations and minor operations may be written with the progress notes, but they should always be headed "Consultation" or "Laryngoscopy," and so forth. Similarly, brief X-ray or electrocardiogram readings may be written or typed on stickers and pasted in, like any other report.

Authorizations and correspondence are, of course, no part of the medical record, but for the sake of convenience they have come to be included. In any situation in which the patient is subject to unusual risk, it is customary for the hospital to safeguard itself against suit by requiring him to sign a witnessed authorization or release. Such releases are commonly secured before an operation, any radiotherapy or hyperthermia treatments, and also when the patient leaves the hospital against advice. A single sheet with printed statements covering all of these possibilities saves handling a number of separate forms. An authorization from the patient is also required before personal information can be given to outsiders. Also, permission from the proper relative must be secured before the performance of an autopsy or the removal by an undertaker.

Correspondence with and about the patient, as well as these authorizations, may be filed separately without greatly detracting from the value of the record. A great amount of special filing is avoided, however, if they are attached to the record. In fact, the inclusion of correspondence may become such a convenience that it will become necessary to sort out letters and cards of a trivial or non-relevant nature and merely note their receipt for the follow-up value. Both authorizations and correspondence are inserted by date. They are sufficiently distinctive in form to prevent confusion and they are convenient thus to the part of the record to which they relate. Operation releases follow their respective operations, and so forth.

Clinic notes are not noticeably different in content or form from the doctors' hospital notes. Both may contain histories, physical examinations, and progress notes and be interspersed with various laboratory and treatment records. The peculiar problem of out-patient notes in a unit record arises when a patient is attending several services during the same period. The hurried clinic doctor must be able to find past notes in his own service readily, but at the same time it should be quite obvious to him what is being done in other departments which may relate to his problem. This dilemma is very neatly met by providing each service with a rubber stamp. This heads all notes with the name of the particular clinic and the date. By this means all notes may follow chronologically regardless of service, and at the same time any particular ones can be found by a quick glance at each page. Furthermore, it is space-saving and cheap, for special forms are not required. So successful is the use of rubber stamps in securing attention and saving time that other uses will doubtless suggest themselves. One stamp calling for a transfer to or a consultation by another service, with space to write the reason, has proved a great help to the doctors and also to the clerical staff who make the necessary arrangements. Diagnoses made in an out-patient service should be clearly marked as such in the margin or underlined, so that they will stand out and can readily be entered on the front unit sheet. They should also conform in their phrasing to the accepted nomenclature, so that they will fit into the diagnostic index without question.

Follow-up notes fall naturally by date among the clinic notes and are readily enough distinguished by a stamped heading. Such a check up on hospital treatments is extremely valuable to the doctor and also to the patient. A complete note usually covers the interval history, physical examination, conclusion as to results, and suggestions for further treatment. When the patient cannot be brought back, follow-up information must be based upon social workers' visits or correspondence. In any case, it is valuable, even if it is merely a notation that the patient was alive at a given date. Brief social service notes of this character or those in any way pertinent to the medical context may appear among clinic notes, provided they are clearly indicated by their stamped heading.

SERIES OF EXAMINATIONS AND TREATMENTS

The recording of those examinations or observations which need to be presented in a series for the sake of comparison or of those treatments which are given as a course over a period of time offer a problem. Obviously, they cannot be entered chronologically without destroying their value. Many of them cover only the period of hospitalization. These on their special forms may be grouped at the end of the progress notes for that admission, rather like a group of tables concluding the chapter of a book.

The graphic chart is undoubtedly one of the most val-

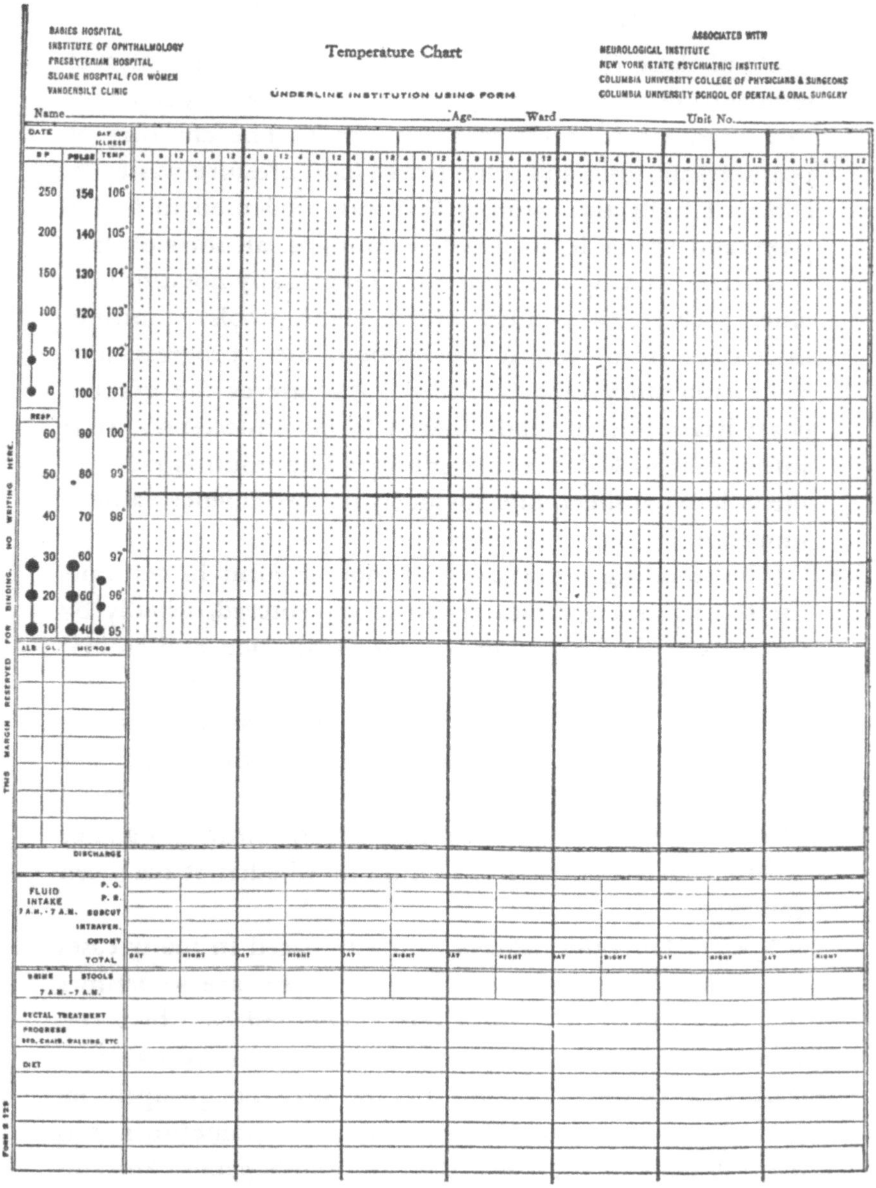
BABIES HOSPITAL
INSTITUTE OF OPHTHALMOLOGY
PRESBYTERIAN HOSPITAL
SLOANE HOSPITAL FOR WOMEN
VANDERBILT CLINIC

Temperature Chart

UNDERLINE INSTITUTION USING FORM

ASSOCIATED WITH
NEUROLOGICAL INSTITUTE
NEW YORK STATE PSYCHIATRIC INSTITUTE
COLUMBIA UNIVERSITY COLLEGE OF PHYSICIANS & SURGEONS
COLUMBIA UNIVERSITY SCHOOL OF DENTAL & ORAL SURGERY

Name_____ Age_____ Ward_____ Unit No._____

DATE
DAY OF ILLNESS

B P	PULSE	TEMP
250	150	106°
200	140	105°
150	130	104°
100	120	103°
50	110	102°
0	100	101°
RESP.		
60	90	100°
50	80	99°
40	70	98°
30	60	97°
20	50	96°
10	40	95°

4 8 12 4 8 12

ALB. GL. MICROS

THIS MARGIN RESERVED FOR BINDING. NO WRITING HERE.

DISCHARGE

FLUID INTAKE 7 A.M.–7 A.M.
P. O.
P. R.
SUBCUT
INTRAVEN.
OSTOMY
TOTAL

DAY NIGHT

URINE | STOOLS
7 A.M.–7 A.M.

RECTAL TREATMENT

PROGRESS
BED, CHAIR, WALKING, ETC.

DIET

Form S 129

Figure 2

GRAPHIC OR TEMPERATURE CHART

uable of these forms. Starting simply as a nurse's interval temperature record on graph paper, it has developed amazingly because it meets so many needs. The charting of pulse, respiration, and sometimes blood pressure was early added. Finally the actual graph was condensed to half a page, and under it, in the date columns, all sorts of data is written, varying with the case. These daily notations include such items as fluid intake, urine, stools, vomiting, discharges from wound, medication, diet, progress, and some laboratory reports. Indeed, this use of the graphic chart has rendered many special forms unnecessary. It is just as easy to follow progress on it. The result is rather a messy looking sheet, but obviously its convenience value is immense.

The standing order sheet is another form in constant use during hospitalization. On it are entered, usually by the nurses, all doctors' orders for medication and special nursing instructions, with the date given and stopped. The data it contains is kept separate from other notes, not only because it may stretch over a considerable period, but also because of its serious character. Whatever the detail of its arrangement, it should be perfectly clear at a glance whether an order is still standing or whether it has been canceled.

Special laboratory sheets, while replaced in many cases by the development of the graphic chart, are sometimes desirable where progress is very closely reflected by a certain test, as for example, blood sugar reports on diabetics. Any special forms of this nature may be grouped together at the end of the progress notes. Sometimes it is a great help to plot such data on graph paper. For this

CONTENT AND FORM

purpose a graph-ruled record sheet without any special heading is adaptable for many uses.

Certain serial therapy records, such as radium or X-ray, have come to be assigned a special position at the end of the entire record. This departure from usual practice was deemed necessary on two accounts. First, such records might easily cover periods of clinic as well as hospital care, and there was thus no obvious place for them in the chronological record. The second consideration was the serious consequences liable to ensue should any prior treatments be overlooked.

SUPPLEMENTARY PROGRESS NOTES

Under this title we include nurses' notes and detailed social service reports. Each of these in its own way is a valuable supplement to the doctors' notes, but each has a distinctive character and both tend to be voluminous. For these reasons it would be most confusing to intermix them with medical notes. They are placed, therefore, each in its own date order, after the graphic charts of each admission. To distinguish them further, colored sheets are used. This makes it easy to find them and equally easy to eliminate these pages, if one is looking for other data.

Nurses' notes have sometimes been regarded as of passing value only and upon the patients' discharge have been either destroyed or put into dead storage. It is quite likely, however, that the real reason for this practice has been the lack of filing space. However that may be, enough has probably been said about the concept of the unit record to make it clear that such an arrangement would be utterly contrary to it. Just because the doctor does rely upon nurses' notes for detail, his own are more concerned with specific problems and do not attempt to give a full picture of the patient's course. As a result, research men frequently find that if their interest does not coincide with that of the doctor writing the record, the nurses' notes furnish the only answers to some of their questions. Bulk can be somewhat reduced by planning the sheet so as to avoid too much blank space.

Social service notes extend the doctors' knowledge beyond the hospital in the same way that the nurses' notes do during his absence. From them he learns the possibilities of after-care, and often they are the sole source of follow-up information. The initial social report follows a fairly standard outline not unlike the doctor's initial examination, covering the reason for the inquiry, a description of the patient, of his household or group, living conditions, financial security, and ending with a summary of the problem and suggestions. At later dates briefer notes indicate arrangements for care, changes in the situation, and so forth, very much like progress notes. In this instance, also, a question arises as to whether these notes properly belong in a medical record, especially since they contain so much of a personal and financial nature. The answer is that they are most convenient and add considerably to the whole picture of the patient. Likewise they are not the only confidential part of the record, so the wisest solution seems to be to include them and safeguard the entire record. Since they are nonmedical, they, too, are made on sheets of a distinctive color. Those concerned with a hospital admission follow the medical notes for it and those relating to clinic care are placed among those sheets roughly by date.

CONTENT AND FORM 27

SUMMARY SHEETS

The third exception to the strictly chronological order of the record is that of summary sheets of any kind. These by their very nature refer to a period and cannot go in strictly by date. Most of them cover the period of a single hospitalization, and so may be placed after the nurses' notes. As a rule, the only one of these to include more than one admission is the "front unit" or index sheet and that of course has a unique place. Any others having a similar range would have to follow it immediately or be placed at the end with the serial treatment records.

A hospitalization summary, or "admission and discharge sheet" on which are collected all the outstanding points of that admission, is practically essential to a unit record. Such a sheet answers most questions about the course in the hospital without the need of searching among extensive working notes. The time thus saved is most appreciated when the patient returns to clinic, especially if a distinctive color makes the sheet easy to find. The following material has been included here.

Admission data, which is similar to the original application data, but brough up to date and adapted to the circumstances of hospital care, is most convenient on this sheet.

The final diagnosis contains in condensed form the conclusion from all the investigation conducted while the patient was in the hospital. It should occupy a prominent position on this sheet and of course conform to the nomenclature used, for the sake of indexing.

Any important treatments performed during the patient's stay in the hospital should be given a similar promi-

BABIES HOSPITAL	ADMISSION AND DISCHARGE SHEET	ASSOCIATED WITH
INSTITUTE OF OPHTHALMOLOGY		NEW YORK STATE PSYCHIATRIC INSTITUTE
NEUROLOGICAL INSTITUTE	If chart is NOT to be used	COLUMBIA UNIVERSITY COLLEGE OF PHYSICANS & SURGEONS
PRESBYTERIAN HOSPITAL	for research, initial here →	COLUMBIA UNIVERSITY SCHOOL OF DENTAL & ORAL SURGERY
SLOANE HOSPITAL FOR WOMEN		
VANDERBILT CLINIC		

PATIENT'S name_____City No._____Unit No._____
                First   Middle   Last

Address - street_____Apt. No._____

   City _____Zone No._____State_____Telephone _____

Former address _____

Circle whether—single married widowed separated divorced—male female   Date of Birth_____Age_____

Occupation _____Religion _____

Birthplace _____Years in U. S._____in N. Y. State_____in N. Y. City_____
                                                                                          L

Race and nationality of parents_____Husband's or wife's name D_____
                   L   L

Father's full name D_____Mother's full maiden name D_____

Location_____Service_____Class_____Adm. Time & Date_____

               Doctor_____

Discharge diagnoses - operations - chemotherapy_____

_____

_____

_____

_____

_____

_____

_____

_____

_____

_____

_____Dr. _____

Additional pathological diagnoses_____

_____

_____Dr. _____

Impr. - Unimpr. - Died - within 24 hrs. - yes no   Follow-up _____Disch. Time & Date_____

Left margin: Blood donor card gives — Yes / No ; Old record sent — Yes / No ; S150

Figure 3
ADMISSION AND DISCHARGE SHEET

CONTENT AND FORM

nence. These would include operations, radium or other important therapy treatments, and anything else which it is desirable to index.

The condition on discharge answers the third important question about a patient, which with the others goes in abbreviated form on the front unit sheet.

A summary on the back of significant findings, treatments, and course fills out the bare outline of the above and supplies any points of special interest on the individual case. Copies of it may go as abstracts to outside doctors.

The signature of the house officer and of the attending doctor on this sheet indicate their responsibility not only for its contents but also for the whole hospital record.

Statistical summaries have developed because careful research men can rarely get all the details they want from past cases. The only way of insuring that they do, even on current cases, is to prepare on a special form a complete list of the items in which they are interested. These can then be filled out with the other hospital sheets, at the time when the data is available. Since they are complete in themselves, they can be temporarily detached from the rest of the record for convenience in tabulating. Suggestions for preparing them will appear in a later chapter.

FORMAT

A plain white record form, or "continuation sheet" is used for the great volume of unit record notes. This practice, in contrast to the employment of separate forms for each kind of note, helps very much to emphasize the continuity of the record. For handwriting it is lightly ruled and is plain for typed notes. Both sides are written on, book-fashion, to save paper and file space. On colored paper the same form may also serve for the supplementary progress notes. This "continuation sheet," like all other record sheets, bears the institution heading. The effect is to give a certain uniformity to the record and an official quality to the notes.

Special printed forms, of course, are clearly indicated for certain purposes, but it has proved wise to use a good deal of caution in adding new ones. In theory, they are very tempting, seeming to offer complete and uniform records with minimum effort, but in practice they are more than likely to prove disappointing. Enthusiasm wanes quickly, and, unless permanent responsibility is fixed in each instance, the stock shelves will soon be filled with expensive and outdated forms. Moreover, too free use of special forms tends to departmentalize the record. In those instances where the need is clear, it is well to experiment for a time with mimeographed copies or rubber stamps, for alterations are almost inevitable in the beginning.

Means of distinguishing various kinds of notes is not limited to special printed forms or titles. Indeed, what the eye really catches is often just the incidental form of the data. This is true of any material, such as an examination which is consistently in outline form, of laboratory report stickers, of any typed notes among the handwritten ones, and of such forms as the graphic chart. Colored paper is effective enough, but too free use of it in anything as long and involved as the unit record tends to become confusing. It has been reserved, therefore, for the supplementary nurses' and social service notes and for the hospital summary sheet. Because these all occupy definite positions

CONTENT AND FORM

among the notes of each hospital admission, they serve as guides to the special notes which uniformly precede or follow them, which thus have no need for a distinguishing color. The first and last places in the entire record, because of their convenience, have been reserved for the most used or most important sheets. Where form or position does not sufficiently distinguish notes, it is always possible to make use of rubber stamps. As already mentioned, these are most effective, as well as simple to use and inexpensive. Colored ink is excellent, too, provided it is possible to use it consistently, as in distinguishing medication from nursing instructions on the "standing order sheet."

Paper and ink assume importance, when one recalls that the record may be in use as long as the patient lives, and even longer for research. Paper with a rag content of 75 percent is not too good, and that of 100 percent is better for summary forms. The 8½ x 11 inch business sheet is probably the most satisfactory, for it permits the use of standard filing equipment. Ink or typewritten notes should be the rule, with the possible exception of carbon copies of pathological reports, if the original is carefully preserved in the department making it.

Covers for unit records must be suited to a great variation in thickness of records, the constant addition of new material, and the hard use of constant handling. The common manila folders soil easily and become brittle rather quickly. Covers made of heavy Kraft paper or jute stock are tough, long wearing, and are still cheap enough to allow replacements when needed. Since, as the record increases in size, the cover usually becomes worn, it is simpler to put on a new one of the proper size than to trouble with expansion folders. By carrying several sizes varying from a single fold to ¾ inch, most records can be taken care of. Those few records which exceed this thickness can be divided into volumes.

A method of binding or fastening these records should keep the material secure and at the same time be quickly opened for the addition of new sheets and also be compact in the files. While the records are being completed it may be necessary to fasten them together with prong fasteners. For permanent use, however, these take up an unbelievable space in the files and make it too easy for sheets to be lost. These difficulties are overcome by fastening the sheets to the back cover with heavy wire staples. The operation of removing the staples with a special tool, adding a new sheet and restapling on a foot machine is much quicker than it sounds. Moreover, because of the machine, it localizes the handling of loose record sheets at one point, where proper care can be taken. When a record is too thick for staples, it may be divided into sheaves, each of which should be stapled separately and fastened into the cover with cloth binding tape.

SUMMARY

A unit medical record aims to present as complete and continuous a story as possible of a patient's medical progress. To this end it contains all the medical data on a given patient, regardless of when or where within an institution it may have originated. If there is an out-patient department, material from there is included equally with that from the hospital proper. To these essential medical notes is added that nursing, social service, or administrative material which rounds out the former or simplifies the handling of the case.

Consistent with the aim of the unit record, this conglomerate material is arranged in chronological order, with exceptions only as demanded by the character of certain data. The first exception consists of any of those examinations, observations, or treatments which are valued primarily in a series rather than individually. The supplementary progress notes of nurses and social workers, because they are nonmedical and often voluminous, are a second exception. Finally, summaries of all kinds clearly cover too much time to fit under one date. However, any of these exceptions which covers a single admission is inserted immediately after the chronological record of that period. Only those which may cover longer periods or are of extreme importance are completely excepted from the date order and placed first or last in the entire record.

Most of the record is written on a uniform sheet carrying no printing except the institution heading. Notes of various types within the chronological sequence are distinguished in a number of ways, as by rubber stamped headings, by colored paper, or by characteristic form. Special sheets for various kinds of notes are used, but only for very good reasons, since too many tend to departmentalize the record. With a very few exceptions, a memorized outline instead of a printed one is preferred, as being much more flexible.

III. MAINTENANCE

IN THE PRECEDING CHAPTER we have seen what a complicated thing a unit record is and how many sources continually contribute to it. From this fact we may very properly conclude that quite a bit of care and planning are needed to keep it up to date and up to standard. If there is a clinic, the problem is especially difficult, for it is impossible to set the record aside for completion following a hospital admission. Actually this period immediately after discharge is apt to see the record in greater demand than usual, by the clinic, by social workers, by anyone corresponding with outside doctors or lawyers, as well as by doctors and secretaries wishing to complete the hospital notes. Failure to appreciate this difficulty, which arises from the nature of the unit record and to plan accordingly is one of the chief sources of trouble in adopting this type of record.

IDENTIFYING THE CASE

The unit record number, especially if it assigned on the patient's first contact with the institution and retained permanently, provides a most convenient identification for everything pertaining to him. Such a sure and simple designation for material is essential to insure its prompt inclu-

MAINTENANCE

sion in the proper record. For this purpose the name alone is far from adequate. Not only are there often several people with the same name, but hasty copying in clinic or laboratory may distort it beyond recognition. Furthermore, since records are usually filed by number, material bearing a name only must be referred to the name index before it reaches the proper record. The use of the number eliminates this step, and when certainty is essential, as on reports, the combination of name and number ensures a high degree of accuracy. In order to obtain the greatest advantage from this means of identification, the number should be assigned as soon as a record is begun and its use advocated as widely as possible. Steps should also be taken to reduce to a minimum two common numbering errors.

Issuance of the same number to different patients can cause very serious confusion, where so much reliance is placed upon the number to designate a case. To avoid this danger a central point to issue the numbers is needed, especially if patients are admitted to the clinic from one office and to the hospital from another. One of the offices or the record department will do. It is not necessary to dole out the numbers one by one. A block of a hundred or so may be issued to each office, and a brief notation kept. At the point where each number is assigned a simple list, or blotter, may be all that is necessary. If admissions are heavy, as they are apt to be in a clinic, it may pay to have record covers, patients' cards, and index cards all stamped in advance with a numbering machine and each set clipped together. This work can be done during slow periods and it prevents the many copying errors which are inevitable when clerks are working under pressure.

Duplicate records for one patient is another error which is very annoying and troublesome to right. Many can be avoided by thorough questioning as a part of the admitting routine. Even with this precaution, however, some patients, either by intent or through confusion, will deny previous care. The best safeguard is a carefully maintained central name index, where every patient has a card, no matter when or how he entered the institution.

PERIOD OF HOSPITALIZATION

The simple addition of one note after another in the bound record, which is the clinic practice, is interrupted when a case enters the hospital. So much new record material of varied character is begun and is in constant use during the entire period that a different procedure for gathering it is inevitable.

The previous record obviously belongs wherever the patient is being treated. Therefore, if one exists, it is either taken to the admitting office with the patient or is called for by that office when it sends for the patient. From there it accompanies him to his floor and is kept conveniently at hand during his entire stay.

New admission data is entered at this time on the "admission and discharge sheet," usually in the admitting office. This sheet then accompanies any previous record to the floor and serves as a nucleus for the new hospital sheets. Some method is also required for distributing this admission data to certain other points in the hospital, such as the information desk, if it is separate, the accounting office, and the record department. There are any number of ways of accomplishing this, varying from teletype or telauto-

MAINTENANCE 37

graph to duplicate copies, or simply the sending of a pedigree card to each office in turn before it is filed for the duration of the patient's stay.

New hospital sheets include, beside the admission and discharge sheet, those for doctors' progress notes, nurses' notes and the graphic charting, and often numerous others, depending upon the service and the case. As these are constantly being added to, studied, and written upon, some kind of holder permitting easy additions and firm support is needed.

On discharge of the patient these loose sheets and the previous record, if there is one, need to go to the record department to be bound together and checked. It is better, with a unit record to have it sent at once, even though the record may not be entirely complete, for it is likely to be in demand very shortly. To insure this with a minimum of trouble, the delivery of the record can be made a part of the discharge routine, possibly the official notice that the patient has left.

ASSISTANCE FOR THE DOCTOR

While the medical profession itself has made all the chief advances in medical records, there is little doubt that the maintenance of these standards puts an increasing and irksome burden on the individual doctor. As a result, hospitals are being asked to increase clerical help more and more. The extent to which they can respond, of course, depends very largely upon the state of their finances. Since most institutions can give only partial assistance, it will pay to consider how this may best be expended.

Typing notes from dictation not only saves the doctors'

time in writing, but it greatly facilitates reference to them. In the latter respect it distinctly furthers the aim of the unit record, for there is little advantage in having material at hand if it is too difficult to read. Since it is usually too costly to type all doctors' notes, the next best thing is to select for this purpose those which receive the greatest use. A list arranged roughly in this order would include the front unit sheet, summaries of each hospital admission, operation, biopsy and autopsy reports, important consultations, X-ray readings, and possibly histories and physical examinations.

Additions to the front unit sheet may occur at any time that a new diagnosis is made in clinic, as well as after each hospital discharge. For this reason it should be detachable, or a special bookkeeping typewriter can be used, which types directly on the sheet while it is fastened in the record. As for the other notes, there are several ways of handling them, each with its own advantages. Dictation directly to a typist at the machine, wherever it can be arranged, is liked because it is very quick. While the use of dictaphones involves an initial cost, it makes it possible for doctors to work at odd hours and for the transcriber to work at an even pace. Dictation to a shorthand stenographer or first writing them roughly himself is about the only way a doctor can get bedside notes typed. The first way is expensive, since the secretary wastes much time waiting for comparatively little dictation. Also no one can share the typing with her or take it over if she is overworked or ill. Copying rough notes does save the stenographer's time and produce a neat record, but it doesn't save the doctor much work.

Convenient places to work are another means of eas-

MAINTENANCE

ing the doctors' record work. If the record department is conveniently located, a study, or several small ones, adjoining it is ideal. Such an arrangement keeps the records close at hand even while they are being worked on, so that it is easy to get them should any be required in the clinic or elsewhere, as they very often are. Since diagnoses are expected to conform to a certain nomenclature, it is only good sense to provide copies of the appropriate nomenclature wherever in the hospital or the clinic cases are being diagnosed. To prevent their thoughtless removal, it is best to have them chained.

Adding miscellaneous material is a clerical job which assumes considerable proportions with unit records. We have indicated how this new material is handled while the patient is in the hospital. There the nurses have the main responsibility, with help sometimes from interns and technicians. It is seldom appreciated, however, how much of this work there is to do at other times. New "continuation sheets" have to be added as those in the records are filled. So also must be correspondence, changes of address, and an increasing volume of laboratory reports, as more and more tests become routine in the clinic. The staple fastening which we have described purposely makes it most difficult to add full-size sheets except in the record department, where the special tools are available. Thus a good share of the work of adding material to the records is automatically centralized, and it seems good sense to go a little further and send all miscellaneous additions there. It is a great deal easier to fix responsibility under this plan, and it may also be possible to schedule this work for comparatively quiet hours when the workers are not subject to much distraction. Both factors contribute to accuracy, and that is an important consideration in this business. An incidental convenience in sending everything of this nature to the record department is that if the record is temporarily out of the file, the new addition may be left in its place in the file to be discovered and added just as soon as the record returns.

MAINTAINING THE RECORD STANDARD

Valuable as this stenographic and clerical help is to the doctors, neither it nor their own good resolve is sufficient to maintain the record standards they themselves set. Some routine scheme of checking is clearly necessary. Fortunately, while a certain amount of professional supervision is needed, a great deal of this work can be handled by a trained lay person.

The lay responsibility for keeping records up to standard very naturally is assumed by the record librarian. Indeed it may be considered her most important function. Hospital notes because of their variety and importance require the greater attention, and the logical time to check them is immediately following discharge, when they are being assembled and permanently bound. Exactly how much detail she is expected to include in this routine examination will depend to some extent upon the requirements of each institution. Some may wish an almost line-by-line review, while others consider it sufficient to cover certain key items only. Surely she should include those essentials of a complete hospital record outlined in the previous chapter and for the most part standardized by the American College of Surgeons and other national associations. In

MAINTENANCE

addition, her training should have familiarized her with the special requirements of the various kinds of cases the records of which pass through her hands.

The conformity of the final diagnosis to the nomenclature is best checked on this occasion also, so that it will fit into the index. It is poor policy, however, to expect this lay person, no matter what her training, to translate inaccurate terms into accepted ones. Much better, if she confines herself to putting the question or making a suggestion to the doctor responsible.

A check slip of some kind is usually placed on the cover while a record is incomplete, for the sake of convenience. It consists simply of a list of those items covered in this examination, with a line for the name of the doctor responsible. Space for a brief question and answer is useful, too. Deficiencies are underlined or checked, so that each man can tell at a glance what he has to do. Also the record librarian need waste no time in reëxamining the whole case.

A current index, or file, of incomplete records is necessary in the record department, for to it belongs the responsibility of notifying individual men of the work awaiting them. If records include only hospital notes, it may be easier to segregate the unfinished records themselves in a separate file, arranged according to the doctors responsible. With unit records, on the other hand, if they are at all active in clinic, this arrangement is very apt to require more labor than it saves. It simply means that a great many cases must be looked for in two places, under their unit numbers and again in the special file. If this is the situation, it is much easier to file the records in their regular place—except when actually being worked on—and to keep a card index of unfinished records. It may be possible to use for this purpose the pedigree card which served in the admitting office while the patient was in the hospital. It already bears much of the information needed, such as the patient's name, number, discharge date, and so forth.

Periodic reports on record deficiencies can also be prepared from such an index by the record department. This is a most effective means of keeping the professional staff informed of the current situation. Since it is difficult to maintain interest in any routine report, however, it is probably better to err on the side of simplicity in drawing these up. Too much detail is apt to discourage a busy man from reading them at all. Sometimes it may help if the record librarian analyzes the material a bit for the staff, indicating any outstanding progress or lapses. Success with this method depends upon her own ability in this line and upon the wishes of the particular staff.

Clinic notes call for much less attention. They are simpler and of necessity far less thorough than those written in the house. There is need, however, for a quick examination of each day's notes to pick up any new diagnoses, if they are to be listed on the front unit sheet or entered in the index. These can be spotted much more readily if the staff form the habit of underlining the terms or of writing "Diagnosis" in the margin. As with final hospital diagnoses, these, too, should be expressed in terms of the accepted nomenclature to permit proper indexing.

Professional responsibility for the quality of the records can never be entirely shifted to a lay person, no matter how capable or experienced she may be. Theoretically, each attending doctor puts his approval on a hospital record—

MAINTENANCE 43

interns' notes as well as his own—when he signs the final summary. Even so, individual members of the staff are bound to differ in their conception of what constitutes satisfactory notes and in the amount of time and attention they give to the matter. Some more dependable and uniform means of assessing the records from the professional angle is clearly needed.

The record committee has been developed to fit just this need. To function effectively, the members need to have a genuine appreciation of the value of records. They should represent the various viewpoints of the staff and should have sufficient standing so that their opinions will carry weight. Men of this caliber are apt to be busy and they can rarely afford time to examine the record of each newly discharged patient. A thoroughly workable solution is for them to review an evenly distributed sample, as every fifth or tenth record, for example. From this they can obtain an adequate idea of the quality of records being written. By taking turns, they can further lighten the burden and still accomplish their purpose. Besides their primary function, this committee constitutes a much needed liaison between the record librarian and the professional staff. By requiring their approval on all new record forms, many ill-considered ones can be weeded out at the start. To them also may be referred the new terms which are continually being suggested as additions to the nomenclature. They and not the record Librarian can best determine which are real disease entities and which just whims. Also, the men on the record committee can accomplish a great deal toward arousing the interest of the rest of the staff in the report of record deficiencies.

MAINTENANCE

SUMMARY

Contained in the unit records is material which under other circumstances would form any number of separate files. Because so much reliance is placed upon them by so many departments of the hospital, it is extremely urgent that they be kept as up to date as possible. The very thing, however, which makes this necessary also makes it difficult, for those records requiring the most work are just the ones in greatest demand. It is most important to appreciate this problem and to plan accordingly. An amazing amount of time can be saved, if the practice is followed everywhere of identifying record material and referring to the records by permanent unit numbers. Whatever can be afforded in the way of clerical assistance and convenient working conditions for the doctors, also, speeds the work of completion. Besides this, the usefulness of the records is increased by having typed those notes which are most frequently referred to.

Maintaining the desired standard for unit records, as for any others, is a matter of systematic checking. While a trained record librarian can attend to the major part of this, it is most important that the distinction between lay and professional responsibility be clearly recognized. To make sure that the doctors carry out their share in practice, as well as accept it in theory, a carefully selected record committee is invaluable.

IV. FILING AND TRANSPORTATION

MUCH OF THE THOUGHT and labor expended in producing good records may be nullified by an inadequate filing set-up. In other words, a thoroughly good record may still be a completely useless one, if it cannot be produced when and where it is needed. Because so much hospital business is concentrated in unit records and because of the clinic demands, the filing situation is utterly different from that in a record department handling only hospital cases. The volume alone is very much greater and also the need for speed, so that all filing considerations assume a much greater importance.

FILING SCHEME

A unified file is not required before unit records are possible. An institution may have unit records while maintaining separate hospital and clinic files, provided that the individual records of patients who have received both types of care are bound together and filed in one or the other of the files. Very often this is the only arrangement possible, because space is not available for a unified file. At best, however, it is a makeshift, involving duplication of effort and frequent confusion. The logical system, once the records themselves are united, is a single file housing all types of records under one numbering system.

46 FILING AND TRANSPORTATION

Accident records and others, which for any reason at all cover only a treatment or two before the patients are sent elsewhere, can likewise be kept in this unified file instead of separately, as they often are. They need not occupy much space, if the application sheets are filed without any covers. The numbers for such cases may be assigned from special blocks, so that they will run consecutively. Then it is possible to file a considerable number of these single sheets loose in one folder, which serves to protect them from the heavier bound records. If, at any future date, one of these cases is accepted as a regular patient, that sheet can be covered as usual and still retain the original number.

The unit numbering system is such a convenient feature of the unit record system that the two things have become confused in many people's minds. An institution which combines under a single permanent number all hospital records of one patient, while allowing him to have a separate out-patient record, does not have the unit record system. Such an arrangement is absolutely contrary to the fundamental concept of the unit system, that of continuing the study of a patient past the period of his bed care: On the other hand, unit records may be filed in any way whatever and still remain unit records, and the institution using them may be said to have a unit record system. Practically, however, numerical filing has replaced all others, because of its greater speed and certainty.

Institutions which do not have clinics sometimes favor the serial numbering system. As each case is readmitted a new number is given, but the existing record is brought forward and combined under the new number with the new record, thereby making it a unit record. The advantage is that active records are automatically kept in the active or new section of the file, and this is a most important consideration where filing space is very limited. In a unified file, however, which contains clinic records, this advantage disappears, for the older sections will still contain a great many active clinic cases which have not been admitted to the hospital in years, if ever. This situation is true to a lesser degree, even where unit records are centered in the hospital file while a separate clinic file is maintained for out-patient cases never admitted to the house. Furthermore, the advantage of a permanent identifying number is lost. People throughout the institution will not bother to keep up with constantly changing numbers. Particularly if there is much reference to the records from the diagnostic index, the permanent number saves tracing many cases from number to number until they are finally found. In general, then, it may be said that unit numbering is best suited to unit records.

Periodic transfers to less accessible storage space is an unpleasant feature of any filing system. Various schemes for weeding out inactive records from the file, thereby deferring the time when a whole section must go to storage, have been tried. The one most often suggested is that of sending all death cases immediately to storage. For study, however, these are fully as valuable as other cases, and often more so. Furthermore, the nuisance of having to look in two files for each order from the diagnostic index quite offsets the tiny percentage of space saved in this way. Much the same faults are likely to be found with any other methods of selecting inactive records. Two files for records in the same number series are simply more trouble than they are worth, almost without exception.

48 FILING AND TRANSPORTATION

The alternative to weeding out is simply to remove to storage, say once a year, enough of the less active end of the file to allow for another year's growth. Among these less active cases there are almost sure to be some which are still coming for treatment or observation fairly frequent. To avoid too frequent trips to the storage room, some special provision must be made for these records. They may be retained under their original numbers in a special file in the main room, or the permanent number rule may be relaxed in their case and new current numbers may be assigned to them. Both arrangements have their drawbacks. In the first, there is the nuisance of two files covering the same series, and in the second, the loss of the permanent numbers. In either case, they will not cause too much trouble, if there are not too many of them—in other words, if records do not have to be sent to distant storage rooms too soon.

Changing to a unified file or to a unit numbering system is best accomplished by starting with all the new cases of a given date. To avoid confusion between identical numbers in the old file and the new, it may be wise to start the new one with a number higher than any yet attained, instead of beginning again with "one." Active cases may be renumbered and filed in the new file, but this is not necessary, unless the old file must shortly go to storage, or unless a change in the form of the records makes it hard to add new notes to old cases. The practice of using a letter with the number for any purpose whatever is to be avoided. It is one of those elaborations which is apt to be far more of a nuisance than a convenience. Six figure numbers are entirely practicable. When a million is reached, it will probably be quite safe to begin again with "one." Even a large

FILING AND TRANSPORTATION 49

hospital is unlikely to have still-active cases bearing low numbers in the first series when the second million is begun.

Reverse numerical or terminal digit filing is an entirely different conception of numerical filing. It completely eliminates the periodic moving of the entire file and, in addition, offers other advantages of equal value.

The system requires the division of the entire active file into one hundred sections from 00 to 99. The records are filed under these sections *by their last two digits*. Thus, the oldest and the most recent records are evenly distributed throughout the room. The manner of subdividing these sections depends upon the size of the file and the number of records desired behind a guide. In a really large file consisting of a hundred thousand or so records the original hundred divisions would each in turn be subdivided into one hundred subsections. For example in the 47 section of the room the guides would run from 00–47 to 99–47. These subguides would refer to the middle two digits of the record number. Finally, back of each of these guides the records would be arranged by their first digits, as 8–00–47, 9–00–47, 10–00–47, 11–00–47, and so on. One hundred sections each divided into one hundred subdivisions mean ten thousand guides for the entire file. If there are 150,000 records in the file, there would be fifteen behind each guide.

In a file which is limited by space to between ten thousand and one hundred thousand records, the original one hundred sections might be divided into ten rather than one hundred subdivisions. The records behind each guide would run something like this: 98–6–31, 100–6–31, 101–6–31, etc. A really small file, less than ten thousand, would need no subdivisions at all.

Advantages appear as one studies and works with this system. Space for growth is made by removing each week or month a number of old records equivalent to the new ones added during the same period. Never does the whole file have to be moved. Also, the entire filing space is used to full capacity all of the time. New guides are never needed except to replace worn ones. A fair division of the file work is automatic, saving supervisory time. Experience has shown, too, that the system brings not only a noticeable increase in speed (since all sections are identical in arrangement) but also an increase in accuracy (since the attention is concentrated on only two digits at a time).

Converting to this system is simple, but it may take quite a time unless considerable empty file space is available to begin with. The process consists of pulling from a straight numerical file all records ending in 01, 02, and so on and arranging them according to the secondary guides. This does not take too long. Only when it is necessary to stop after pulling out a few numbers in order to condense the old file and thus free more space does the conversion job become long and tedious.

SPACE AND HOUSING

Adequate filing space in a convenient location is a prime need for any record system and one which has very rarely been properly recognized. With the unit system, however, this requirement assumes such importance that the lack of it alone may prevent the adoption of the system. If an institution has an active clinic, it is essential that a unified file (or even any file containing unit records) be located convenient to it, for by far the greater part of the circulation will be

FILING AND TRANSPORTATION

there. As a corollary, there must be sufficient space in this location to accommodate the records until the great majority become inactive. Just how many years this will take depends upon the institution, but it is pretty apt to be more than at first assumed. It is quite likely that a far from negligible proportion of clinic cases may continue active for ten or even fifteen years. This point at which out-patient cases become practically inactive is probably the best measure of the active filing space required.

The arrangement of an active file of this size begins to assume importance. If the file is a straight numerical one, placing the active end near the main exit will save countless steps. If clerks are working at desks in the same room with the file, it will help to separate the two as much as possible, so that those working at the files do not need to brush past those at the desks or talk over their heads. If artificial light is needed for much of the work, it is wise to consider the type furnished. Anything which helps to reduce glare will save a good deal of misfiling and consequent annoyance and loss of time.

Storage space, even for records ten or fifteen years old, should not be too remote. Not only will there always be some patients unexpectedly returning for care, but there is apt to be quite a bit of correspondence and research on cases dating back as far as twenty-five or thirty years.

In housing medical records thought must be given to maximum use of floor space, convenience, protection of the records, and cost. Because vertical files keep the contents both clean and accessible, they have largely replaced the book shelving used when records were bound in large volumes. In view of the universal problem of space it is surprising how often four- rather than five-drawer cabinets are used. Even though the latter cost more, twenty-five per cent more filing capacity is worth considering. In a straight numerical file, especially if clinic records are included, the higher numbers are much more active than the rest. Consequently, the best equipment is desirable there, even if it cannot be afforded throughout. A reverse numerical file, of course, is equally active throughout. If there are no loose sheets, filing the records folded side up in the drawers will save time and prevent misfiling, for each file then appears as a unit, rather than as a number of separate sheets.

Shelving especially designed for medical records has been developed and deserves serious consideration. It eliminates many of the disadvantages of the old volume shelving and achieves some remarkable savings in floor space and is more convenient than vertical filing. This type of shelving consists of panels approximately thirty inches wide, nine shelves high, and completely enclosed at the back and sides. Since the records are filed on their long edges, the shelves are only ten inches high, over all. Thus a girl of average height can reach eight shelves without a stool. Active records are kept on shelves three, four, five, and six, numbering from the floor, which can be used without either squatting or stretching. These four shelves are open for greater convenience and speed and depend upon constant use to keep dust from accumulating. Shelves one, two, seven, and eight hold the less active cases. These and the ninth shelf (for storage only) are all closed with simple covers. Four movable dividers on each shelf keep the records upright even when the shelves are not very full. The same panel with covers for all the shelves is suitable for storing records.

Filing the records lengthwise not only puts more shelves

FILING AND TRANSPORTATION 53

within reach, but it also reduces the frequency of aisles. The saving in floor space, as compared with vertical files, is considerable. A large installation may house as much as seventy per cent more records in the same area, even if only eight shelves for active use are compared with five-drawer files. The cost even when made to order should not exceed that of good cabinets. If standardized, they should cost much less, being so much simpler in construction.

Microphotography offers an attractive solution to the problem of ceaselessly accumulating records, but it should be studied from all angles before it is adopted. For unit records, roll film would be suitable only when their use for patient care or research has become negligible. By that time, however, it is questionable whether the cost is warranted.

Specially reinforced floors are of the utmost importance wherever any number of files are to be accommodated. A filled five-drawer file will weigh close to a quarter of a ton, and this is concentrated on about three square feet of flooring. Architects make their specifications accordingly. The danger comes later on, when a change of location is proposed and attention is focused on every consideration except this hidden one.

REQUISITION-FILLER SYSTEM

Although unit records are used by so many departments and individuals in a hospital, they must be produced at once whenever the patient appears for care.

The requisition-filler was developed to simplify and speed the pulling out and finding of records in a file. It is simply a blank slip of cheap paper or light card of a size to be easily read at the file. Anyone wanting a record writes close to the top—the slip being used narrow edge up—his name or office number, the date he wishes the record, and the record number. Clinics can use their date stamps for this purpose and so need write only the numbers. One slip is required for each record, so that as each one is pulled, the slip may be put in its place. Since it is just long enough to extend a trifle above adjacent records, the information, being near the top, is easy to read. There is no comparison between pulling records with this combination requisition-filler and pulling them from a list, stopping each time to make an entry on an out-card. When the record returns to file, the filler may be destroyed, for re-use usually involves more labor than it is worth.

A tabbed variation of the requisition-filler is convenient when records are being sent out singly instead of in groups. The tab is simply an extra inch and a half in length, separated from the rest by perforations. The name of the person or clinic calling for the record is repeated on this tab. Then when the record is pulled the tab is easily detached, to be clipped to it as a label indicating the destination. Such a detail may appear trivial, but the accumulated time it saves is worth while.

A return system is very necessary to make certain that records, removed from doctors or offices upon the patients' attendance in clinic, are sent back promptly and without fail. This may be effected almost automatically and without any special bookkeeping by taking advantage of the requisition-fillers. When a record called for is out of file, the procedure is to draw a line on the new requisition just below the date on it and to copy under this line the information from the filler in file. With this addition the new

FILING AND TRANSPORTATION

requisition now tells not only who wants the record, but also where it can be found. A messenger may be handed several such requisitions without further instructions. As soon as each record is secured and sent to its new destination, the new requisition becomes a filler replacing in file the old one, which is destroyed. Now, when the record is returned to the record department for filing, the line on the filler which she is about to remove indicates to the file clerk that that record must be sent back to the place it was taken from—unless this notation has been entirely scratched out, implying that its return is not wanted. If it is to be returned, the clerk merely crosses out the data above the line and adds the current date. This leaves the place from which the record was secured alone on the filler, and the record goes back there at once.

Transfer cards were developed to keep track of records moving from one part of a busy clinic to another, without unnecessary red tape. Some patients may visit two or three services and in addition be interviewed by social workers or administrative officers, all in the course of a single day. At each point their records are needed. The labor involved in making out a new filler at each transfer, of getting it to the record department and filing it there is considerable. Furthermore, most of it is absolutely wasted, for in only a very few instances is there any occasion to trace these records. Therefore each clinic has its own transfer card. This is simply a card about the size of the records, ruled and divided into three columns. On it are entered, each day, the number and destination of every record leaving that clinic. It is thus a very simple matter to trace the few cases which require it. Likewise, if these cards are returned to the rec-

56 FILING AND TRANSPORTATION

ord department at the end of each day, the clerks there can make a second use of them. For the information of each clinic, they may note the numbers of all cases requisitioned but not sent and state very briefly where they may be found or what is being done to find them.

TRANSPORTATION OF RECORDS

Even if the record department is located to the greatest advantage, there still remains a considerable problem in transporting records in such continual demand. If a new building is in prospect, it will pay to look into the possibilities of a pneumatic tube system or the endless chain carriers used in some large libraries. These are expensive, however, and each has disadvantages as well as advantages, so that careful study of the individual problem is indicated. If such devices are out of the question, messengers must be used, and there is much to say in their favor. They can do a great deal beside just carry the records.

Record bags, in which to carry a number of records, are not merely a convenience, they are just about indispensable. A very satisfactory and inexpensive one may be made to order as follows: Two stiff covers—¼ inch Masonite does very well—a little larger than the records, are fastened together by a six-inch strip of strong duck extending across the bottom and about two-thirds of the way up the long sides. A card holder attached to one side holds any desired label and one inch webbing handles make it easy to carry. Because these bags collapse when empty, they do not require much storage space.

Trucks for handling larger number of records will save time and strength in countless ways. Any carpenter can

FILING AND TRANSPORTATION

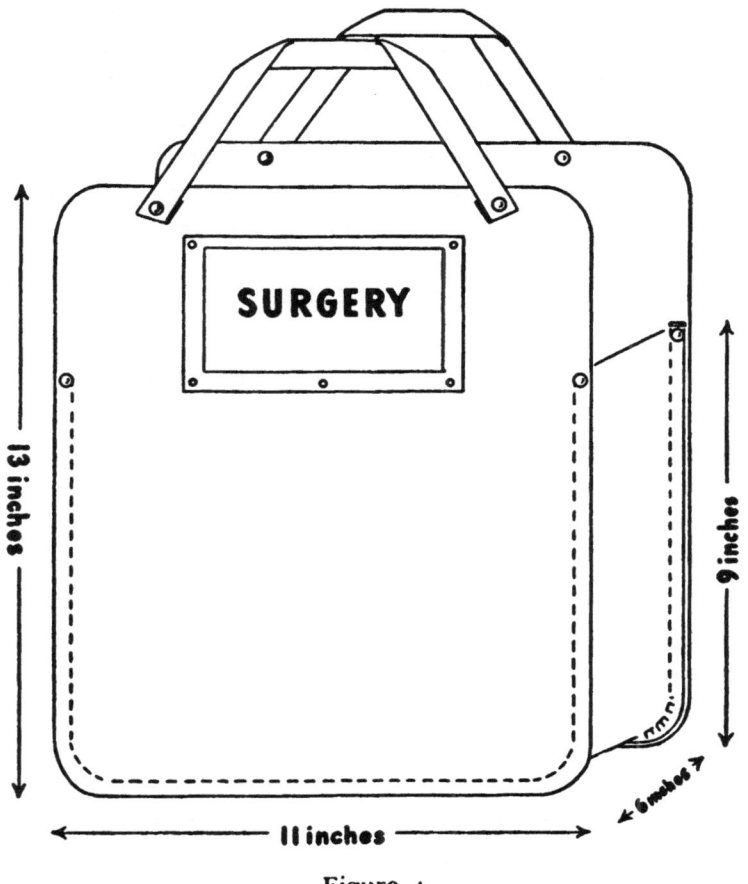

Figure 4
RECORD BAG

make them. Good inside measurements for the body are twelve inches wide, six or seven inches deep, and twenty-eight inches long. This should be mounted on legs raising it to desk height and equipped with castors large enough to permit it to be rolled on and off elevators easily. Three partitions will prevent the records from falling flat when it is partly empty. If these are also removable, such trucks can be quickly converted into sorting bins. By placing them—either with or without castors—beside the desks, the clutter and annoyance of stacks of records disappears completely. It is like working from a movable file drawer.

FILING SCHEDULE

In facilitating the pulling and filing of records, the arrangement of time is nearly as important as that of space and equipment. Some operations may have to be done over and over again, just because they are done out of the logical order.

The daily return of active records to the record department is just about a necessity with cases of this kind. Exceptions may be made for doctors working on groups of cases, for certain offices, or wherever else a very good reason exists. Nevertheless, the bulk of those out to clinic and to social workers need to come back and be filed daily. On first thought, this may appear to involve unnecessary labor where records are required again shortly. It is the easiest way, however, to get them to others who need them in the meantime and to add any new material promptly. Actually, a great many cases may be handled routinely in the department in less time than it takes to run down a few scattered ones.

The order of work within the record department should likewise follow the proper sequence, to avoid needless duplication. There are obvious advantages in doing the filing as quickly as it comes in. Nevertheless, if the volume is

FILING AND TRANSPORTATION

considerable, both time and misfiles will probably be saved by reserving it all until the end of the day, when the majority of the records are returned. At this time, when the rush of the day is over, it is possible to work without interruption on filing alone. Doing the job once instead of at half a dozen times saves time, and concentrating on it alone saves errors. Large institutions have found it worth while to have a special evening shift to do the filing and, with it, to attend to the addition of miscellaneous material.

Once this is finished and everything is in its place again, records which have been ordered in advance may be pulled with a minimum of tracing. If there are many of these, owing to the appointment system in a large clinic, a night shift to perform this work may be advisable. This arrangement leaves the files free during the day for nonappointment and miscellaneous calls. It incidentally keeps the department staffed at all times to handle emergency calls. Such extensive arrangements are not needed by a small hospital, of course, but a slight adjustment of clerks' hours may accomplish the same thing.

SUMMARY

The circumstance, that clinic notes form a part of unit records, makes the problem of filing one of utmost importance. Because many clinic patients continue to attend for years, a very much larger active filing space is needed than is usual for hospital records alone. Furthermore, the daily calls from the clinic itself, or from social and administrative offices associated with it, constitute all but a small fraction of the demand for records. Because this is so, it is absolutely essential that the main files be closely connected with the clinic, either by location or by some rapid transportation system.

The concentration of data in unit records multiplies the demand for them throughout the institution, in addition to the volume of clinic calls. Because of this, problems of filing and transportation require very careful attention, with due regard to the peculiarities of each hospital. One principle has always been found sound under a variety of applications. It is that of centering everything possible pertaining to a record in its place in the numerical file. The use of a permanent number identifying that place for every possible reference to the record is one instance. This practice saves untold time because it is so direct. The requisition-filler system, which concentrates information about the record at this point, is another. Similar to this is the practice of leaving all additional material in place of the record when it is out. Both methods eliminate separate little files and lists and save a clerk from having to look in two places. Likewise from this experience has grown the dislike for separate active and inactive files covering the same series of numbers. One cannot tell beforehand in which place the record will be. In line with this principle, too, is the insistence upon the daily return of active records to file. It brings them up to date and puts them in position to meet the next call promptly.

V. INDEXING

NO OTHER TYPE can compete with a numerical file for speed and simplicity, but in itself it is utterly incomplete. There must be indexes to unlock the material stored there. The absolute essential, of course, is a name index. Then, in order to use the records for study, there must be at least a diagnostic index also. To these two basic ones may be added elaborations or minor indexes as the requirements of each institution dictate. Indeed, no index should be conceived of as an end in itself, but rather as a convenience or tool. The closer it can be fitted to actual daily needs, the better.

NAME INDEX

Before attempting to decide upon the details of the name index, it will help to consider, first, exactly what purpose it is intended to serve. Should we be able to obtain from it all the most important facts of each record, or will it be enough, if we are just directed to the right record with certainty? There may well be circumstances where the more complete information is really needed. Experience suggests, however, that the number of trips to the record file which it may save is likely to be far outweighed by the time consumed in adding the extra data to thousands of cards.

INDEXING

The index which we are about to describe has just one aim, that of identifying each patient quickly and surely. The reason for stressing this function of the index in a unit system is because it is the only way of insuring unit records, if patients do not choose to admit previous care.

```
┌─────────────────────────┐  ┌─────────────────────────┐
│         681470          │  │ Med    2/28/42  8/14/48 │
│ Doe, John         33y   │  │ Surg   8/20/42  9/3/42  │
│ John              Mary  │  │                         │
│ M    W    S       NY    │  │                         │
│ 333-W-144-84-NY         │  │                         │
│ 1901 Broadway NY        │  │                         │
│                         │  │                         │
│              Laborer    │  │                         │
│ Adm Em   7/10/42        │  │                         │
│ 8345                    │  │                         │
└─────────────────────────┘  └─────────────────────────┘
         Front                         Back
```

Figure 5

NAME INDEX CARD

The name card, for such a purpose, is stripped of all nonessential data and it is designed to be read at a glance. It is a common practice to employ cards which have served elsewhere during the patient's hospitalization. The intention, of course, is to save copying. As so often happens in trying to adapt an instrument to more than one purpose, it ends by being imperfectly suited to its major function. In this instance, the result is to clutter up a permanent card with data of temporary value. Copying, here, is justified by the time saved in referring to an index of simple and uniform cards. Also, it should be remembered that cards for pa-

INDEXING

tients attending only the clinic will have to be made out anyway for the index and that these are usually in the majority. What is considered essential will vary with conditions, but the following items have stood the test of time very well.

Name   Age   Record number
Father's first name   Mother's first name
Sex   Race   Marital state   Birthplace
Address
Occupation
Service and date of first contact with the institution
Service and dates of each subsequent hospitalization

By abbreviating the items of the third line and reserving the back of the card for those of the last line, all this material may be typed upon a standard half-size card (2¼ x 3 inches) without the slightest crowding. There is even space for several changes of address. This is possible because these few items require no printed titles to mark their places on the card, merely light ruling to guide the eye. Such a card does not have to be read; a glance or two is enough. Its superiority over even a 5 x 3 inch card in this respect is apparent when the two are seen side by side. The value of typing rather than writing the front of these cards is obvious, but it is hardly worth removing a card from the file merely to add new admission data on the back. The use of a pen at the files is much quicker and quite as satisfactory, since this part is not so frequently referred to.

The physical set-up of the name index should include the best rag stock for the cards to insure their permanence. They need also to be flexible enough for easy typing. Nothing else yet offered competes with the vertical steel card file for housing this index. Half-size cabinets are available as standard equipment. If in any way possible, the drawers should neither be too high for easy reading nor too near the floor, for they will be in constant use. A second and equally important advantage of the small cards appears in the compactness of the index. It occupies just half the usual space.

As for the scheme of the name index, it is clear from the description of the card that one per patient is all that is needed. The addition of a new one on each admission accomplishes nothing except to consume space. Likewise in disfavor is the practice of starting a new index every year or so. This is a plain nuisance, with nothing in its favor. The tremendous state and business indexes in successful operation should reassure any hospital which fears its index will become unwieldy. There are also satisfactory ways of limiting the size when that becomes absolutely necessary. It is not too much, however, to allow for a unified in- and out-patient index covering twenty-five years or over. Many patients live and are fully capable of returning during this period, and without a continuous index old records are easily missed. The reason for combining clinic and hospital cards in one index is much the same. It is the best guarantee against duplicate records.

The best arrangement for a name index is something which firms specializing in business methods have been seeking for years. To look into their developments is only good sense, although careful study of individual conditions should precede the adoption of a system. To balance skepticism regarding anything new, it is important to recognize the fallacy of assuming that the strictly alphabetical arrangement is the simplest, merely because it is the most familiar.

INDEXING 65

In dealing with English spelling, especially in a population which is adapting foreign names to English pronunciation, the alphabetical index is very far, indeed, from simple. The inevitable variations in spelling may scatter what is really the same name very widely. Even experienced file clerks cannot be sure they have thought of all the possibilities. Where this situation prevails, thought might be given to some system based upon sound rather than upon spelling.

The maintenance of this index is most important, for it is the one place in the institution where every patient is recorded. Only the most experienced and careful clerks should do the filing. Also, if it is to be fully depended upon, cards of new patients need to be filed very soon after their admission to clinic or hospital—in other words, soon after their unit numbers are assigned. The practice of waiting until discharge or even, as some do, until the hospital record had been completed, before filing the name card, destroys much of the value of the index. Changes of name or address need to be made upon the name card as well as upon the record, for they are most necessary in fixing identity. Very helpful, too, is the free use of cross-indexing for any patients using more than one name or even for variations of the same name.

Doctors' introductory letters received before the patients appear can be a nuisance, even if there are not many. They should be attached to the new records before the first doctors see them, but even a daily check will not accomplish this. It is easy, however, to put the patient's name on a specially colored card and file it. Just as soon as one of these patients is received and his name is checked or his regular card is filed, this special one will be caught, indicating that a letter is waiting.

Admission and discharge lists are prepared daily in most hospitals. Provided they carry the numbers as well as the names, they can form a very handy supplement to the name index. Quite often someone will not remember a patient's first name and possibly not the last one accurately; yet they may have a fair idea of when he was in the hospital. In such instances, it is much simpler to find the number on these dated lists. Inexpensive binders preserve them and keep them in order.

DIAGNOSTIC AND TREATMENT INDEX

As with the name index, it is a good idea to have in mind what this diagnostic and treatment index is to accomplish, before studying it in detail. Here, too, opinions differ as to whether it should be simply an index to the records or whether it should also do double duty as a source of statistics. Simple counts in answer to specific questions can be made in any case, but to plan on obtaining routine statistics of any value in this way seems futile. Definitions vary too much with the disease, with the type of institution, and with the purpose of each study. It seems better—at least until the subject of morbidity statistics is somewhat further clarified—to look upon this primarily as an index to the records, a means of collecting those having certain similarities. To accomplish this satisfactorily requires a careful study of the kind of demands which must be answered and their frequency. Indeed, no detail of this index should be adopted or long maintained without weighing the labor involved against the need it will meet. There is probably no other

INDEXING

part of record department work where it is so easy to squander time in fruitless procedures.

The card for the diagnostic and treatment index is not nearly so standardized as is the name card. Different forms, even within the same index, may be desirable. The size is unimportant, except that the smaller standard sizes

I 1			LOBAR PNEUMONIA		
1/41			**3/41**		
512011.111	M56	1010	537097.053	M52	1018
536706.019	M52	1016	256065.019	F44	1018
536661.053	D F56		538090.215	M79	1010
450693.019	M31	1010	532166.215	F26	
530910.019	F46		524163.187	M55	1017
529425.004	A F68	1018	369538.121	M31	
			538336.262	M52	
			514989.016	D F58	1010
2/41					
289832.175	M53	1016			
562627.175	F28				
644827.052	M45	1017			

Figure 6

DIAGNOSTIC INDEX CARD

are probably easier to handle. Whatever the form, it should be easy to read. This implies typing and the arrangement of all entries in columns. This provision allows the eye to run rapidly through many cards, picking out easily just the details required. As with the name cards, printed titles may well be eliminated where they are not really needed.

As for entry data, the absolute minimum is the record number. Unwanted records may sometimes be eliminated at the start, if, in addition, each entry indicates the attending doctor (by number to save space), and the patient's sex and age. A "D" or an "A" to mark a death or an autopsy is helpful, as is some means of distinguishing private cases from ward cases, if different rules apply. Instead of giving the date of discharge with each entry, it is usually enough if the entries are made by month, and so headed. Details of diagnosis or treatment which do not warrant separate cards may be preserved as descriptive items on the more general cards. Columns of this type occupy very little space, if the nomenclature provides a numerical code with which to express them. In a similar fashion, each of several diagnoses may be entered as complications of the others. This last possibility, however, is apt to take up a good bit of space and time and it is most unlikely to be much used. All of the other items can be typed on a single line—even on a half line, if they are numerically coded and the card is wide enough—as follows:

Month and Year

Record No.   Doctor   Death   Sex   Age   Diagnostic detail
             or   or
             Service Autopsy
               (Private cases in red)

The physical set-up of the diagnostic index should be of the best quality, for this index, too, will be used for years. Indeed, a span of twenty-five years is often desirable to contrast treatment methods or to test their effect by long survival periods. This index will not grow as rapidly as the other, for instead of one card for each patient, a good many discharge entries are made on each card. For housing it, nothing seems really superior to the simple vertical or horizontal file. Expensive and long-wearing printed guides

INDEXING 69

may be bought, but plain tabbed ones, on which the headings can be typed, will do very well. In fact, they have the advantage of flexibility should new divisions or combinations be desirable as the index grows or the requirements change.

The scheme of this index in its simplest form requires an entry to be made under each separate term—be it diagnosis, treatment, or symptom—by which the record might be called for. If the doctor has written on the "admission and discharge sheet" three final diagnoses, a symptom, and an operation, this record number and its accompanying data will be entered in five places in the index. Symptoms and treatments, of course, might be regarded as diagnostic detail and entered as such with each of their associated diagnoses. However, since surgeons are apt to request all cases having certain operations, and diagnosticians all those showing certain symptoms, separate entries for these seem indicated. An exception may be made in the case of obstetrical entries, where there are so many descriptive details related only to this type of case. By making one long entry of all, they can be found easily, and much time is saved. While it is quite feasible to have a separate index for diagnoses, one for symptoms, and another for operations or treatments, there seems nothing to recommend it, and a certain amount of duplication can be saved by combining them in one index. Likewise, it is easier to keep hospital and clinic terms in the same index. As they are usually asked for separately, the entries can be made on different colored cards.

The arrangement of this index very naturally follows that of the nomenclature used. If none has been adopted, an alphabetical index may be set up, but the best that can be said for it is that it is better than none. Synonymous terms tend to scatter cases of the same disease throughout the entire index. If a staff have agreed to pool their experience in the form of records, one of the most necessary steps is the adoption of a uniform language for cataloguing the records. To prepare a terminology is such a tremendous undertaking that most hospitals simply accept one already in use. Only one, at present, offers any representative opinion or provides for periodic revisions, and this one we shall shortly describe in detail.

The maintenance of the diagnostic index does not imply promptness so much as a little planning. As each case usually calls for several scattered entries and as unit records are continually on the move, it is a great deal easier to work from cards than directly from the records. Hospital pedigree cards, which are removed from the index of incomplete records as the cases are finished, will serve very well, with the simple addition of the final diagnosis and any operations performed. Clinic diagnoses, with the date and record numbers, can be copied on scratch paper or cards of the same size. With the data in this form it is possible to accumulate common terms and make a number of entries at the same time on each index card. Terms which have been suggested for addition to the nomenclature sometimes constitute a minor problem. Those due to new medical discoveries are apt to be in demand, and yet there may be a long delay before it is finally decided just how they are to be added. If they are entered on temporary cards, distinguished by color or flags and placed as near as can be determined to their proper place in the index, they will be available during the

INDEXING

interim. When the decision finally is made, they can be properly filed.

THE STANDARD NOMENCLATURE AS A BASIS FOR INDEXING

As a basis for the diagnostic and treatment index the *Standard Classified Nomenclature* has several distinct advantages. As we indicated in the first chapter, it has a certain authenticity, derived from its representative character and its permanent organization. On this account it has been widely adopted, with the result that doctors in different hospitals who are interested in the same problem have far less trouble than they once had in collecting comparable cases. The consistent emphasis upon etiology which characterizes this nomenclature very much simplifies the work of assembling records upon that basis. Finally, the numerical code shortens the operation of the index in many ways.

The basic plan of the nomenclature needs to be clearly in mind before the arrangement of the index can be understood. It is usually referred to as a dual classification, indicating that each disease is described both by its anatomical location and by its etiology. There are twelve major anatomical divisions and thirteen primary etiological categories, one of which provides for diseases of undetermined cause. For greater exactness, each term is numerically coded. This number is hyphenated, the first part always indicating the location of the disease and the second its etiology. Most terms are coded by three anatomical and three etiological numbers, but fine distinctions in either part of the code may require the use of four to six digits. The x and y which appear are the result of attempting to suit the code to punch-card tabulation. Standard tabulating cards allow for twelve holes in a column, designated commonly by the ten digits and x and y.

Of course the *Standard Nomenclature* suffers the disadvantages as well as the advantages of such wide variety of opinion. Because each specialty requires the finest distinctions in its particular subject, the book is large, and it seems to demand more detail in making a diagnosis than is possible for anyone but a specialist. Actually all it requires is the statement of such details as are known and the classification of the rest as undetermined.

Manifestations or symptoms are distinguished in the *Nomenclature* from disease entities. Since it is so often desirable to index the former as well as the latter, they are included in the book, but in supplementary lists. They, too, have code numbers, but these are simple arbitrary numbers, without all the anatomical and etiological connotations. These lists are offered as suggestions to which each hospital may add whatever it desires to index in the way of laboratory tests or symptoms. It is emphatically stated, however, that these supplementary terms by themselves cannot constitute the diagnosis of a case, but merely its description. One of the regular terms must accompany them, even if it is only "undiagnosed disease."

There are some manifestations which occur so widely or are of such importance that a more convenient means of designating them is needed. Among these are abscesses, sinuses, scars, cysts, and a good many others. These are indicated by adding to the etiological code a decimal and a digit. Certain of these digits are quite consistent in mean-

INDEXING 73

ing throughout the book, while others vary with the etiological category and some are entirely arbitrary.

The Nomenclature of Operations is correlated with that of disease by using the same anatomical code and by replacing the etiological symbol with one signifying the type of operation. By this arrangement one book provides all of the most desired ways of classifying and indexing a case, by diagnosis and also by major symptoms and treatments.

In constructing an index upon the Standard Classified Nomenclature—or upon any other, for that matter—it is important to realize how different in purpose are the book and the file. The former aims to provide a term for every recognized disease. Whether it occurs commonly or is extremely rare makes no difference. Likewise it allows for all the fine detail which a doctor requires in describing the individual case. For these reasons, thousands of titles must be included. In the index, on the other hand, only a few hundred terms will be outstanding because of their frequency or because they are the subject of much study. In calling for records for study, doctors commonly, although not always, use broad general terms. Because of this great difference in viewpoint, a good deal of adjustment is called for in setting up the index. This may be made in a number of ways. The following is merely one which has worked well.

The anatomical plan of the Nomenclature very naturally suggests the basic arrangement of the index. We have seen, however, that the twelve main groups are somewhat arbitrary, being limited by the number of holes in the column of a machine tabulating card. As a result, such unrelated things as mental diseases and regional injuries are brought together. To avoid this, it is a simple matter to break up several of these main divisions in a manner more in line with the actual relationship of the diagnoses included. The list which follows suggests twenty-three anatomical divisions as the primary ones for the whole index. They are lettered for convenience in referring to them.

ANATOMICAL DIVISIONS

A	Psychobiological unit	(00.–)
B	Body as a whole	(01.–)
C	Regions	(02. to 0x.– excl. 04. and 06.)
D	Abdomen and peritoneum	(04. and 06.–)
E	Skin	(10. to 18.–)
F	Breast	(19.–)
G	Bones, joints, bursa, ligaments	(20. excl. 208 209 21. to 26. 2x.–)
H	Muscles, tendons, fascia	(208 209 27. 28. 29.–)
I	Respiratory system	(3. .–)
J	Cardiovascular system	(4. .–)
K	Hemic and lymphatic systems	(5. .–)
L	Mouth and throat	(61. 62. 63.–)
M	Other alimentary organs	(60. 64. to 67.–)
N	Liver, bile passages, and pancreas	(68. 69.–)
O	Urinary system	(70. to 74.–)
P	Male genital system	(75. 76.–)
Q	Female genital system	(77. 78.–)
R	Obstetrics	(79. 7x.–)
S	Endocrine system	(8. .–)
T	Nervous system	(9. .–)
U	Eye	(x1. to x6.–)
V	Ear	(x7. to x9.–)
Y	Undetermined system	(y. .–)

INDEXING

The etiological categories make very satisfactory subheads under each of these main anatomical divisions. As they are consistent throughout the index, they seem easier to remember and less confusing than further anatomical divisions at this point. In this respect, also, a modification of the classifications of the Nomenclature seems desirable. The number of headings, however, are reduced by combining some of the less distinctive ones. It has proved convenient to put the symptoms and operations relating to each anatomical system after its etiological divisions, as separate divisions. The secondary guides of the index, therefore, appear as follows:

ETIOLOGICAL GROUPS, SYMPTOMS, AND OPERATIONS

0	Diseases due to prenatal influence	(–01. to 09.)
1	Diseases due to infection (higher and lower forms)	(–1.. 2.. excl. late effects)
3	Diseases due to poisons	(–3.. excl. late effects)
4	Diseases due to trauma or physical agents	(–4.. excl. late effects)
5	Late or secondary effects of disease	(–5.. 7.. and late effects)
6	Diseases due to unknown cause	(–6.. 9.. x..)
8	New growths	(–8..)
Y	Undiagnosed disease	(–y..)
	Symptoms	
	Operations	

Common or important specific diseases may be given their own guides under the etiological divisions. This final

76 INDEXING

breakdown is the one which will vary with the type of hospital. It is purely for convenience and may be altered at any time to meet changing circumstances. It is very helpful if

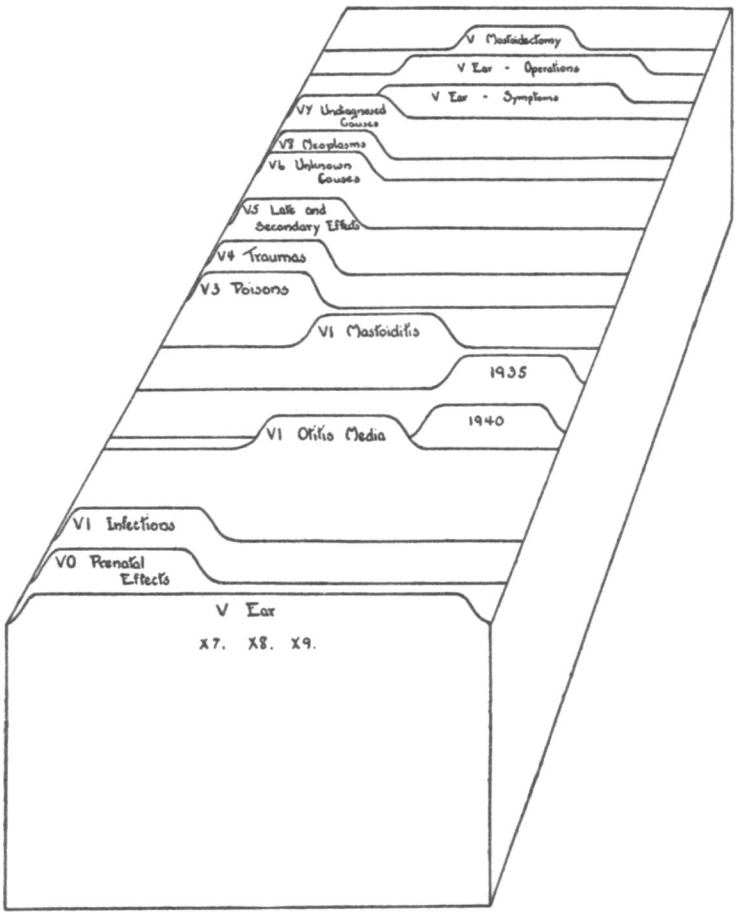

Figure 7

SECTION OF DIAGNOSTIC INDEX

INDEXING

the disease is named, as well as indicated in code, on these guides. Sometimes a single term in the *Nomenclature* is thus separated, as measles. In other cases the term may be more inclusive, as sinusitis. In this latter instance the particular sinuses and microörganisms in each case are entered on the cards as diagnostic details. In the same way all the miscellaneous conditions, which do not rate a special guide, are entered together under each etiological guide, as, for instance, respiratory infections or neoplasms of the respiratory system. This arrangement of the index makes it very easy to get out general groups of cases, and it still remains easy to run the eye down the columns of diagnostic detail and select any refinements given in the original diagnosis. It is all preserved.

SECONDARY INDEXES

In addition to the two essential indexes, the operation of any given record department may call for secondary working indexes. We have already mentioned one for incomplete records, arranged according to the doctor responsible. Either as a part of this or separately it may be desirable to maintain a record of all the cases treated by each man. As with the diagnostic index, the data included should be determined after careful consideration of the use which will be made of them and they should be reviewed from time to time with actual experience in mind.

Microphotography of old indexes is an excellent solution when they are still required for reference but occupy too much valuable space. From 3,000 to over 8,000 cards can be photographed on a 100-foot roll of sixteen millimeter film, depending upon the card sizes. This fits into a box

1 x 4 x 4 inches. On a special viewer, or reader, the negative image appears full size again. To attach a roll and find a given card is nearly as quick an operation as finding it in the file. It is not extremely expensive, either, for the photographing equipment may be rented for the duration of the job and the viewer alone retained permanently. Moreover, any careful clerk can do the work without special training.

SUMMARY

More than almost any other part of the record set-up, the indexes need to be planned to fit the individual institution. The tendency toward overelaboration needs to be guarded against, especially with the diagnostic and treatment index. Every detail of content and arrangement should be weighed against the actual demands, and occasionally reweighed to meet changing circumstances. The arrangement should aim to draw together as far as possible those things which will be required together, whatever the subject of the index. Guide cards can be very helpful, if their titles are obvious and do not necessitate reference to a book for their interpretation. Legibility of the cards is highly important in every case. Typing, the elimination of useless printing, careful spacing, and, where possible, a columnar arrangement are all important factors to this end.

VI. RIGHTS, RESPONSIBILITIES, AND SAFEGUARDS

THE STATUS of any medical record is extremely hard to define. It has at least three distinct functions and by its very nature involves the rights and responsibilities of several different parties. What is more, the position of these parties is shifting continually with changes in medical practice and with developments in social welfare. Many hospitals, too, are forced to maintain distinctions between ward and private records. Far from simplifying this situation, the unit system aggravates it in practice because of the wider demands it places upon the individual case. Anyone responsible for medical records is repeatedly called upon to make decisions—often minor but sometimes very important—involving all these different aspects of a record. Before attempting to suggest any general rules, therefore, it may pay to consider various functions of the record and the positions of the principal parties.

FUNCTIONS OF THE RECORD

As an individual medical document the record fulfills its primary purpose. As such it constitutes the sole written evidence of the main business of the institution. This is true in any case, but with a unit record this phase does not end when the patient is discharged from the hospital. It recurs every time he comes back to clinic for a treatment or a check up. On this account, because there is such frequent conflict between this and other functions of the record, it needs to be generally recognized that this use takes precedence over all others.

The conception of the record as a basis for medical study and research is responsible for most of its development. Although this function of the record may be temporarily suspended to allow for further care of the patient, it is probable that in the long run it is fully as important as the other and that it may be more so. At any rate, the value of the record for study needs to be fully appreciated, and care should be taken not to hinder this use unnecessarily.

The incidental use of the record for the personal affairs of the patient confronts the hospital administration with a considerable problem. Not only do such demands consume a far-from-negligible amount of clerical time, but the complications of litigation often render the proper safeguarding of these records extremely difficult. Such demands cannot be dismissed, because often this is the only source of information of great value to patients. Furthermore, the hospital itself frequently has an interest in the collection of insurance or of other claims to cover unpaid bills.

POSITION OF THE PARTIES CONCERNED

The patient, by committing himself for medical care, invokes responsibility in the doctor and likewise in the institution to do everything possible for his care. Institutions have repeatedly been held legally liable in cases of gross neglect. Originally the medical record was seldom thought of in this connection. As records have become increasingly dependable, however, the idea is emerging that to provide an adequate record and to keep it available is part of the institution's undertaking toward each patient. The business of furnishing an outside doctor or another hospital with medical information, which has long been regarded as a courtesy arrangement, may have a sounder basis in this conception of it as a duty toward the patient. In regard to private cases, where the doctor still retains a greater share of responsibility, the institution's part may be a little less, but it cannot be entirely avoided, and everything indicates that it is increasing.

The patient's right to privacy calls for constant alertness on the part of those responsible for his record. In order that a person may speak freely to his doctor—as to his lawyer or his priest—information imparted under these circumstances has long been given special legal protection as a "privileged communication." Medical ethics provides the chief safeguard, and hospital administrations and employees tacitly accept this view when they enter into a working partnership with the medical profession. In actual practice, however, it is extremely easy to confuse this confidential nature of the record with other considerations. Especially is it important to realize that without the patient's consent, no friend or relative, no matter how close—unless he be a legal guardian—is entitled to confidential information from the record.

The patient's limitation with regard to his record likewise prohibits his own access to it or to medical data from it, except as approved by the doctor. Should he wish to use it for such personal business as collecting insurance or legal damages, he may find also that the hospital has a right to provide for an outstanding bill before accommodating him.

The doctor, as we have seen, assumes a certain responsibility for the content of each record when he signs his name to the final diagnosis or summary. In him, too, resides the authority to decide what the patient should be told about his condition, and also what relatives or others need to know, to insure proper care of the patient. This is part of professional responsibility and no lay person is entitled to assume it.

Each doctor's access to his own records for study offers no problem, so long as he does not remove them beyond reach, should any of his patients require sudden care. The practice of making all ward and clinic records available to all members of a hospital staff is general wherever the doctors of an institution work as a staff and share their experience. Patients have no occasion to object, because the whole staff look upon this as confidential material. There is also a very old understanding that when patients receive all or part of their care free, anything which may be learned in the course of their treatment may be used anonymously for the advancement of medical knowledge. Private patients, who pay the doctor as well as the hospital, are in a somewhat different category.

The state on certain occasions may override the rights of the patient and demand his record as legal evidence. In most instances in which he is claiming compensation or damages this contradiction is more apparent than real. His very action in bringing such claims implies his consent to

FUNCTIONS

the use of any evidence which will support them. In criminal actions, of course, this is not so often true.

The use of medical records as a source of public health studies is a growing one and it is still not clearly defined. The reporting of births, deaths, and communicable diseases is an unquestioned requirement of the state, but to what extent and under what circumstances records from private institutions may be used for public studies is not quite so clear. Usually, appreciation of the purpose of the work produces free coöperation, especially if those handling the records are well qualified and responsible.

The position of the hospital administration—as may have already become apparent—is very largely one of responsibility to each of the other parties. Although it, rather than the patient or the doctor, owns the record, its use of it is limited to securing certain statistics therefrom or to withholding it occasionally until a patient signs a lien in the case of an unpaid bill. On the other hand, there is the growing tendency to transfer from the doctors to the hospital more and more of the responsibility for satisfactory records. Also, in addition to its proper business of supplying records for the care of its patients and the studies of its staff, the hospital must undertake to furnish whatever data is required in connection with the personal affairs of their patients.

SAFEGUARDS WITHIN THE INSTITUTION

To assure the records' availability at all times is the primary purpose of regulations within the institution. This necessarily implies *that records be kept consistently within* *the walls of the hospital.* Once assurance has been obtained that records can be found readily, however, it is too bad to hinder the doctors' use of them by any unnecessary restrictions.

To preserve the records from those who have no right to see them is the object of nearly all the other hospital rules. The chief danger arises when an employee becomes a patient or is the relative or friend of one. Because of their knowledge of procedure it is not always easy to thwart the attempts of such people to obtain improper access to records. That it may be done thoughtlessly quite as often as with guilty intent does not lessen the risk. The record librarian and her assistants usually find it sound practice to question any call for a record which is not obviously in line with routine business. In cases in which this is difficult to determine, it helps to require permits from instructors or department heads. Where it is suspected that attempts may be made to obtain a certain record, it may be necessary to entrust it to someone in authority or at least to fasten a note to the outside cover stating that it should not be given out without special permission. A distinctive label on the cover is likewise needed if special rules apply to private records. The identity of a person asking for a record may occasionally present a problem, if the hospital has a large courtesy staff. The usual hospital uniform is a help, but it sometimes happens that further identification, such as a prescription blank, must be asked for. In any event, record clerks should be impressed with the need to establish identity before giving out a record or information, no matter what unpleasantness may be incurred, and they should be assured of administrative backing in the matter.

FUNCTIONS

DEALING WITH OUTSIDERS

Safeguards in dealing with outsiders have as their main aim to prevent information from reaching persons unentitled to it. The practice of requiring a notarized authorization from the patient before giving out information from his record is the best single protection. Such authorizations should really be read, however, and not merely accepted on the assumption that they are correct. Of course, in transferring patients directly to other institutions or in correspondence with the referring doctors no such precautions are indicated. In fact, any correspondence with *known* institutions or doctors is reasonably safe. Telephone calls for urgent information can usually be verified by calling back after checking the number. Beside the requests for detailed medical reports, there are numerous inquiries from schools, courts, employers, and others which require merely enough information to account for absence of individuals from duty. Usually the patient asks for the statement himself, so that his consent is clear. Even if he does not, his authorization is rarely needed unless a diagnosis is required. If it is and if it might be detrimental to the patient, it should be ascertained that his doctor has explained it to him, and he should be required to sign a release. Otherwise the certificate should not be issued.

To withold nonpertinent data from those entitled to certain specific information is a second consideration in giving out medical information. This offers a more difficult problem, especially in litigation cases. There the temptation may be very great to use some detrimental but nonrelevant bit of the patient's history to influence the case. The safest rule, except as the law clearly requires otherwise, is never to give the record itself into the hands of an investigator. Instead, some responsible person should answer from the record whatever questions are required. Exceptions to this rule may obviously be made for investigators from public bureaus or for outside doctors who have been properly vouched for and approved by the administration.

Among other helpful practices is that of consistently withholding the names of doctors and nurses. These individuals can always be produced, if really required, but ordinarily they have little to contribute and should be spared the bother of needless questioning by insurance men or lawyers. A great convenience is the hospital's own proof-of-death form for furnishing this data to insurance companies. To use this familiar form saves time and it also provides a carbon copy for the record. In sending for information from other institutions, a good deal of delay can be avoided by making sure that patients' names are given accurately and if possible are accompanied by a little more identifying data. The exchange of medical information intended for the patients' care is all looked upon as a part of hospital business, and consequently no charge is made. Information supplied for the personal business of the patient is another matter, and it is customary to charge a small fee, although really important data is not withheld, even if the patient cannot pay for it.

Responsibility for handling all this outside business is usually given to the record librarian. This may often be the only possible arrangement, but it is surely far from ideal. Even with experience and what help she may obtain from a busy house staff, she still lacks the medical judgment

FUNCTIONS

to handle correspondence with professional men in any but a routine manner. This problem assumes special importance when many patients are referred to an institution by doctors who are not members of the staff. To such a man, a letter from another doctor dealing with the particular problem of his patient means vastly more than a mere transcript of hospital care. Such individual treatment inevitably raises his regard for the institution. Where such relationships are important to a hospital, it may pay very well to put the responsibility for this business upon a retired doctor or one who is otherwise unable to practice.

Compensation and litigation cases, likewise, warrant special attention, since they are such a valuable source of income to the hospital. To the record librarian, who so often carries the responsibility for them, they are very apt to be just an annoying interruption to her regular work. Where a hospital expects to collect from these sources, it may pay to assign this business to someone connected with the financial office, who can give it the attention it deserves. Such a person would make a systematic effort to learn of all new cases through clinic registrars, the admitting or credit office, the accident service, and so forth. He would keep a simple file of current cases, keep informed of the status of their accounts, and make certain that all possible collections are being made. He would prepare reports for the compensation commission and for lawyers in liability cases and handle subpoenas for such records.

SUBPOENAED RECORDS

The matter of subpoenaed records warrants some attention, as they consume so much time and are so often the object of sharp practices likely to violate the patient's rights. The problem of the patient's consent does not arise, since it is either implied by the action or is overruled. The difficulty comes from the desire of lawyers to obtain the records before trial in order to prepare their cases. That they have justification in this demand is no doubt true, but fear of unscrupulous use of nonpertinent data causes many hospitals to refuse. As a consequence, lawyers commonly attempt to obtain the records by issuing subpoenas considerably in advance of the trials. In such cases, the records need not be produced until the day of trial. The simplest check on this is the court calendar, published in the *Law Journal*. Opinion as to when a subpoenaed record should be handed over to the lawyer ranges from turning it over at once on reaching court to withholding it until the case is about to be called, or even until the record is sworn in as evidence. Nothing but an order from the judge can compel the hospital to give it up before it is sworn in, but hospital messengers are repeatedly subjected to trickery, intimidation, and bribery in attempts to secure earlier access to records. This is another reason why this business is best handled by some responsible person whose principal concern is these cases. Such a person, too, can swear to the validity of the record, should it be admitted as evidence. Unless it is impounded by the court, when it remains under the court's protection, it should be brought back to the hospital at the end of the day. If it is required a second day, a new subpoena, including fee, is necessary. In the event that the hospital is the defendant, it is wise, of course, to have the hospital attorney look over the record or any information from it before it reaches the patient's lawyer.

FUNCTIONS

Compensation cases are a much simpler matter. On subpoena they go to the office of the commission, and may safely be left there as long as required, for the commission is a disinterested party which appreciates the value of hospital records.

SUMMARY

So varied are the functions of the medical record and so divergent the interests of those concerned with it that to regulate its use properly calls for a thorough understanding of the rights and responsibilities of each party involved. Most of the difficulty, however, arises from the confidential nature of the record. Most safeguards are required on this account, whether dealing with those within the institution or those outside it. While not essentially different from any other record in this respect, the unit record tends to raise issues more frequently because it includes material of value to so many different people and is consequently subject to a greater number of demands.

VII. SOURCE MATERIAL

HALF THE VALUE of unit records comes from their unique qualifications as source material for study and research. Certainly this purpose was conspicuous in the minds of those who originally conceived the unit system. Nevertheless, this concentration of data on each patient, fundamental as it is, is only the first step in any study. The care of a patient in all of its aspects produces a great conglomerate of observations. Out of this must be collected those pertinent to the study in hand. Next, these selected items, from all the cases comprising the study, have to be tabulated. Finally, the resulting tabulation requires analysis and evaluation. Of these four stages in research, the first, that of making the original observations, is included in producing the record itself. The last, analyzing and evaluating the results, belongs to the subject of statistics. Therefore we shall concern ourselves here only with a manner of collecting data which has proven well suited to the unit record and with methods of tabulating such material.

OUTLINING THE STUDY

Defining the study may seem superfluous, but actually it is the most essential step in the whole undertaking. To undertake research with only a hazy idea of what it is to accomplish may come close to complete failure. At best it will necessitate frequent revising of forms and reworking of the material. It is practically impossible to foresee all exigencies, but the more thought expended at this stage, the smoother will the rest proceed.

The purpose of the study needs to be stated in so many words. Is it to weigh the effectiveness of a new treatment or test against the currently accepted one? Is it to discover those factors which contribute most toward infection or death in a given diagnosis or treatment? And so on. Sometimes there may be several questions in mind, but too broad an inquiry is less likely to be successful. Merely the vague accumulation of all sorts of data about a given kind of case is not apt to be worth the effort. When a question does arise about it, it is so often found that just the detail needed to answer it has not been included.

A rough survey of possible material may avoid later disappointment. Quite often a doctor finds that certain observations which he himself always enters in a record with special care are only intermittently recorded by others. This situation is practically inevitable in research studies which go into great detail and attempt to extend back over a number of years. Because of it, doctors frequently have to relinquish the idea of basing their studies on past records and are forced to set up a plan for collecting what they want from current cases. The statistical summary sheets mentioned in a previous chapter were devised for this purpose—to insure the inclusion of all the required detail at a time when it is available.

The unit of the study is another thing which should be clearly in mind from the very first. Most often one has to decide whether it is to be the patient, the admission, or the disease, test, or treatment. It obviously depends upon the subject and the purpose of the study. As soon as the unit has been settled, some plan is needed for handling such exceptional cases as present duplication in any respect. For example, an obstetrical study which includes the result to the infant must make some allowance for cases of twins.

The criterion, like the unit of study, is determined by the purpose. Clear definition is essential here. If leaving the hospital alive is the measure of success, it is rarely correct to assume that every death is a failure, for some are usually due to causes quite unrelated to the particular study. Classifications must be provided so that such cases can be eliminated or assigned to the proper category at the beginning of the tabulation. Sometimes following a treatment long lists of symptoms or tests are required, to evaluate success or failure. If this is so, a summary classification is needed without too many groups.

The variants to be tested by the criterion may be different treatments, tests, personal characteristics, or even lists of symptoms or laboratory findings made before a treatment.

Qualifying factors present much the same type of items. The only difference is that one knows beforehand fairly well how the qualifying factors will effect the results, while the effect of the variants is the question to be answered by the study. For example, the study aims to determine which is more effective in treating a certain type of cancer, radium or surgery. These two treatments, probably broken down into more detail, are the variants. The length of time between the discovery of the first symptoms and the treatment

```
BABIES HOSPITAL
INSTITUTE OF OPHTHALMOLOGY                                              ASSOCIATED WITH
NEUROLOGICAL INSTITUTE              SURGICAL SUMMARY                    NEW YORK STATE PSYCHIATRIC INSTITUTE
PRESBYTERIAN HOSPITAL                                                   COLUMBIA UNIVERSITY COLLEGE OF PHYSICIANS & SURGEONS
SLOANE HOSPITAL FOR WOMEN                                               COLUMBIA UNIVERSITY SCHOOL OF DENTAL & ORAL SURGERY
VANDERBILT CLINIC
```

1-6 7-9	NAME _____ OPERATING DATE _____ UNIT NO. _____
10 11 12	SEX male female RACE white negro yellow other AGE _____ RISK good fair bad
13-14	DIVISION 1st 2nd Fract. CLASS ward private DATA sufficient insufficient
15-17	DOCTOR OPERATING _____
20	ASSISTANT _____
21-27	DIAGNOSIS ON DISCHARGE _____
28-32	OPERATION _____
	OTHER OPER. SAME TIME same incis. _____
	other incis. _____
	TEACHING VALUE yes no ANESTHETIST nurse md PREOP. DIAG. ESSENTIALLY CORRECT yes no

	PREOPERATIVE COMPLICATIONS	37		(41)	
33			1 Vascular—arteriosclerosis	8	Preoperative shock
0	None	2	thrombo-ang. oblit.	9	Prev. oper. during this adm.
1	Cardiac—hypertension	3	Raynaud's Disease	Y	Other preop. complic.—specify
2	arrhythmia	4	phlebitis		
3	decomp.—past or present	5	varicose veins	42	MOUTH HYGIENE
Y	other—specify	6	hemarthrosis	Y	Good
		Y	other—specify	X	Fair
34		38		0	Bad
1	Respiratory—cough only	1	CNS & periph. nerves—arteriosclar.		NUTRITION
2	asthma	2	tabes	1	Obese
3	bronchitis	3	paresis	2	Medium
4	bronchiectasis	4	psychosis	3	Thin
5	tuberculosis	5	alcoholism	4	Emaciated
6	upper respir. infection	6	periph. nerve trauma—sensory		ANESTHESIA
7	emphysema	7	motor	5	Intravenous
Y	other—specify	Y	other—specify	6	Inhalation
35		39		7	Spinal
1	Genito-urin.—congenital malformation	X	Skin—infection of foot	8	Local
2	obstructions	0	other infections	9	Other—specify
3	infections	1	necrosis—ulcer		
4	nephritis	2	abrasions or burns	43	PREOPER. MEDICATION
5	nephrosis	3	lacerations	0	None
Y	other—specify	9	Abnormal bone condition	1	Morphine
36		40		2	Barbiturate
0	Alimentary—peritonitis	1	Metabolism—diabetes	3	Avertin
1	peptic ulcer	2	myxedema	4	Atropine
2	gastritis	3	hypothyroidism	5	Scopolamine
3	jaundice	4	anemia—primary	6	Anesthesine
4	diarrhea	5	secondary	Y	Other—specify
5	ascites	Y	other—specify		
6	cirrhosis	8	Generalized syphilis	44	DURATION OF OPERATION
7	obstruct.—paralytic	9	Pregnancy	1	1—29 minutes
8	mechanical	41		2	30—59 "
9	constipation	1	Any prev. oper.—regional	3	60—89 "
Y	other—specify	2	abd.—transverse	4	90—119 "
		3	vertical	5	120—149 "
		4	muscle—split	6	150—179 "
		5	hernia	7	180—239 "
				8	240—299 "
				9	300 min. and over

Figure 8
SAMPLE STATISTICAL SUMMARY FORM

45	SUTURE MATERIAL	50	WOUND HEALING	56	
0	None	0	No complications	1	Vascul.—phlebitis
1	Silk	1	Infect.—trivial	2	infarct.—pulm.
2	Cat gut	2	stitch abscess only	3	regional
3	Silver	3	serious	4	hemarthrosis
4	Steel	4	Skin separation	Y	other—specify
5	Dermal for skin	5	Hematoma		
Y	Other—specify	6	Necrosis	57	CNS & Peripheral Nerves
		7	Hemorrhage	1	disorientation
46	FIXATION OF BONE	8	Disrupt. of wound without evisceration	2	cereb. thromb.
0	None	9	" " " with "	3	hemorrhage
1	Suture	X	Fistula	4	palsy, central
2	Metal	Y	Other wd. healing complic.—specify	6	periph nerve trauma-sensory
3	Connective tissue			7	motor
4	Bone	Z	No wound healing	Y	other—specify
5	Plaster	51	POSTOPER. COMPLICATIONS		
6	Kirschner wire	0	None	58	
Y	Other—specify			X	Skin—chemical burns
		1	Cardiac—coron. occlusion	0	physical burns or abrasions
8	Tourniquet	2	arrhythmia	1	decubity
9	Lane technique	3	decompensation	2	other—specify
		Y	other—specify		
47	INCISION			4	Metab.—intract. diabetes
0	None	52		5	thyroid storm
1	Regional	1	Respiratory—cough only	6	other—specify
2	Abd—upper—transverse	3	bronchitis		
3	vertical	4	pneum.—lobar—clin.	7	Postoper. hemorrhage
4	muscle split	5	x-ray	8	Postoper. shock
6	lower—transverse	6	broncho—clin.	9	Succeeding oper. during this adm.
7	vertical	7	x-ray	Y	Other postop. complic.—specify
8	muscle split	8	atelectasis		
		9	lung abscess	59	TRANSFUSION, ETC. (at any time)
Y	Intestinal intub.—Miller-Abbott tube	Y	other—specify	Y	Phage, intravenous
48	CLOSURE	53		X	R. B. C.
0	Layers—undrained	1	Genito-urin.—retent.—function.	0	Plasma
1	drained—subcutaneous	2	organic	1	Whole blood
2	intraper.	3	traumatic	2	Fresh citrate
3	extraper.	4	cystitis	3	Stored blood
4	other wounds	5	pyelitis	4	Other, specify
5	Thru' and thru—undrained	6	catheterization		
6	drained—subcutaneous	7	anuria—cardiac		DEATH
7	intraper.	8	renal	5	Death credited to other oper.
8	extraper.	Y	other—specify	6	None
9	other wounds			7	Due to operation
X	Tampon	54		8	Due to postoper. complication
Y	Other—specify	X	Peritoneum—peritonitis	9	Other death
		0	subphrenic abscess		
49	DRAINAGE	1	other abscess	60	PREOPER. DAYS IN HOSPITAL
0	None	2	ascites		(incl. day of op.)
1	Cigarette	Y	other—specify	Y	Emergency operation
2	Rubber tube				
3	Penrose	4	Aliment.—stomatitis	61	POSTOPER. DAYS IN HOSPITAL
4	Tampon	5	tonsillitis	Y	Transfer from other service
5	Packing	6	parotitis		
6	Rubber dam			62	POSTOP. DAYS TO ONSET OF COMPLIC.
Y	Other—specify	55		Y	Same day
		0	nausea		
8	Aspiration of joint	1	vomiting	63	
9	OPER. IN TREATMENT ROOM—specify	2	distant.—relieved by rectal treat.	Y	Chemotherapy
		3	ileus—paralyt.—clin.		
X	BREAK IN TECHNIQUE—specify	4	x-ray		SPECIAL DRESSING
		5	mechan.—clin.	1	Phage dressing
		6	x-ray	2	Zinc peroxide
		7	jaundice	9	Other, specify
		8	diarrhea		
		9	hiccough		
		Y	other—specify		

Figure 8
SAMPLE STATISTICAL SUMMARY FORM
Reverse of form

SOURCE MATERIAL

is a qualifying factor. In less specific studies, this distinction is not so obvious and the two tend to merge.

A listing in detail of all the items, whether they be criteria, variants, or qualifying factors, is essential before any form can be prepared. It is not enough to say "Admission Symptoms;" one must list all those which may pertain to this study. In dealing with amounts of any kind—temperature readings, days of care, fluid intake, and so forth—it is necessary to decide whether they are to be treated as exact measurements or are to be fitted into a scale of ten or more classifications. Should a patient, for instance, who was in the hospital seventeen days be listed in this way, or is it enough to indicate that he was there between sixteen and twenty days? To answer this, it is necessary to consider how it is to be presented in the tabulation.

PREPARING THE FORM

Drawing up the form for collecting the data is not such a task, once this foundation has been laid. If there are comparatively few items, a card may be filled out for each case. These are easy to handle, but for an elaborate piece of research they are not big enough. For this, the letter or record-size sheet is most convenient. Indeed, it is the only size to consider if the study concerns current cases, for then it forms part of the record, at least temporarily. Very detailed studies may even require a folder. Where there are so many items on a page, it is very much easier to read if they are arranged in either two or three columns, possibly headed by the patient's name, number, and other brief identification, and pedigree data. Spacing in general is extremely important, on sheets which are so full. A crowded-appearing sheet is enough to discourage anyone from filling it out. It is also easier to fill out the form, and to check it, too, if the items follow the logical time sequence of the case.

Since the details are listed, not much writing is required, but under each heading it is wise to leave space to write in any item omitted from the list. It is also very sound practice to provide under each heading such a term as "none" or "not stated." This makes it clear at once whether nothing was stated or whether this group was overlooked in filling out the form. If a tabulating method requiring a code is to be used, a great deal of time can be saved by putting the code number immediately before each item. Then, in filling in the form, it is necessary only to circle the number to indicate the occurrence of that item. Even if an amount of some kind is to be fitted into a classification, it is wise to provide a place in which to write it when given, for then the checker can make sure that it is included in the proper group.

INSURING COMPLETION OF FORMS

To insure the proper completion of such elaborate forms requires preparation. Even if one doctor is to do all the work himself, it is a good plan to have someone check the sheets after him to pick up little careless errors which are almost bound to creep in. For this checking of details, trained clerical help is apt to be better than another professional man. Such help is especially needed, if the forms are being filled in by men who are not directly interested in the study. Not only must each sheet be examined for omissions and contradictions, but someone must make sure that a sheet is obtained for each case.

SOURCE MATERIAL

TABULATING THE MATERIAL

Tabulating, as well as checking the forms, offers a qualified lay person an opportunity to assist in research. Both types of work, however, call for frequent consultation with the doctor who is conducting the study. This is especially true of the tabulating, for as it proceeds new relationships are revealed and questions arise which may suggest quite different lines of inquiry than those at first comtemplated. Many of these a lay person would miss, because he lacks the necessary special knowledge.

Of tabulating methods there are several, and it may pay to examine briefly the possibilities of each.

The large sheet, on which one line represents an entry and the various columns the items to be tabulated, is one of the commonest. It is a way of collecting data as well as of tabulating it. If there are not many items, it serves very well as a running record from which totals may be accumulated. It is not well suited for correlating the various items, however. It is too hard on the eyes to attempt much of this.

Written work cards, which may be sorted and tallied in any desired arrangement, offer a much more flexible method than the sheet. By it certain groups of cards may be sorted and studied in more detail. Also, if routine daily or monthly tabulations are made from the cards, annual reports may be totaled without handling too many cards at once. For any considerable volume of cards, however, hand sorting is inadequate.

Cards which come with holes punched all around the edges offer a very neat solution to this problem. The occurrence of an item is indicated by cutting out to the edge the hole which represents it, using a little desk punch machine. By this device large quantities of cards can be sorted for specific items very rapidly. With long slender needles the cards still having a certain hole intact are lifted out, leaving the ones which have had that hole cut out and which accordingly possess the given characteristics. Counting is usually done by hand, although machines are made to do it, if the volume of work warrants it. These holes are standard four to the inch, but the cards may be obtained in various sizes, thus allowing for more or fewer items. Since finer distinctions can be written on the card, this method of tabulating will accommodate a fairly detailed study. It is better adapted, however, to less elaborate studies than most medical researches.

Machine tabulating cards offer the best means of correlating these hundreds of details. These provide twelve holes in a column and there are eighty columns on the standard card. Originally developed for the handling of census material and since then adapted to large-scale bookkeeping, the possibilities of this method are endless. There are machines to punch the cards numerically and also in alphabetical code, others to sort the cards, tabulate them, calculate and print the results, and to perform many other incidental operations. Although such methods may seem on too vast a scale for an ordinary hospital, there are ways by which they may be made available without too great an outlay. First, there is the possibility of coding the material in the hospital and sending it to a service bureau to be punched and tabulated. This is not very expensive, but it is obviously suited to regular reports rather than to special studies, in the course of which new questions are continually arising. It is far more satisfactory to have the basic machines, a simple punch and a card counting-sorter, which may be rented for a fairly small sum. By using with these a special multiple code, devised especially for this purpose, and a calculating machine, it is possible to add amounts very quickly, as well as to sort and count the cards.

The use of machine tabulation for comparatively few but very elaborate cards is a special development. Most machine set-ups are intended for just the opposite purpose, to handle great volumes of fairly simple cards. Even with careful checking of the summary sheets, some are so elaborate that contradictory items are occasionally overlooked. These cause considerable trouble if they get into final tabulations before they are discovered. To avoid this, it may prove worthwhile to make a preliminary run of the cards, making sure that columns intended to total do so and watching for any obvious errors in sense.

The form of the tabulations depends upon the material and is really a subject for statistical discussion. Study or advice along this line will help in this respect, as well as with the evaluation of results.

OTHER TYPES OF STUDIES

Beside the elaborate research studies which have been the subject of most of the preceding discussion, there are several other types for which records do or might form the basis.

Administrative studies are commonly limited to statistical or financial reports, drawn from sources other than the records. It would seem desirable to correlate with these items the various diseases treated, which, after all, constitute the real business of the hospital. Some such thought probably lay behind the old practice of listing the number of cases under every single diagnosis entered in the index during the year and publishing it as an annual report. This is not only a terrific job, but it is almost valueless. For reference the index itself is superior, and general trends which might help in administrative planning are quite obscured by the detail. To comprehend morbidity experience from the administrative as from any other viewpoint, the data should be presented in the form of a morbidity list. This gives emphasis to important diseases, it groups closely related ones, and it lumps together the minor ones, so that the total number of titles is not beyond the mind's grasp. If such a list is in general use, so much the better, for comparisons between institutions can be more easily made.

The service analysis of records, which aims to acquaint the members of each professional group with the quality of their own work, is surely one of the most valuable uses of the records. While it may not be strictly research itself, it poses many questions which require the more thorough type of investigation to answer. It was this function of records, also, which directed the attention of the American College of Surgeons to their importance in raising the standard of surgical work. In their concern they suggest a sheet tabulation of the monthly experience of each service, showing the number of cases, deaths, infections, and many similar details indicative of success or failure. Such reports can be prepared by the record librarian, to serve as a basis for discussion at staff meetings. Of course any other method of tabulating can accomplish the same purpose.

Outside requests for statistical data constitute rather

a problem. For one thing, compliance with such inquiries frequently consumes considerable time. In such cases, it may pay to ascertain something of the standing of the individual or organization. If this does not call for doing the work on a courtesy basis, it is not unreasonable to make a fair charge. This will not only weed out the idly curious, but it permits some clerk to prepare the material on her own instead of hospital time.

A far graver problem arises from the fact that so many individuals and even some organizations lack the experience or training to compile dependable statistics. There are plenty of pitfalls in this work under the best conditions, but when material is assembled from a number of different sources they are greatly multiplied. Lack of precise definition is the chief trouble, and comparisons are made, in quite good faith, which are completely misleading and untrue. If it is impossible to refuse to supply data which one suspects may be mishandled, the best thing is to send with it a statement of just how it was obtained. It is often necessary to stress the kind of hospital—whether it takes all comers or refuses chronic or contagious diseases, whether it maintains an ambulance or includes a maternity or children's service. All such factors influence the incidence of any disease and the death rates. For example, the death rate from coronary heart disease will be lower in a hospital which treats children than in one which does not, unless a correction is made. Even the counting of cases of a given type is not simple. It should be indicated whether readmissions and interservice transfers are included or not. These merely suggest the errors which may occur from carelessly gathered data.

SOURCE MATERIAL

SUMMARY

Valuable as unit records are as medical source material, it still requires hard thought and planning to secure from them all that is needed for a careful piece of research. Material for such studies is usually best obtained from current rather than past records, because in the case of the former summary sheets which are part of the record insure the collection of all needed detail. The success of this method depends, first, upon a clear definition of the aim of the study, and also upon a plan to insure the completeness of the data of each case. For this purpose clerical assistance is desirable, such individuals being usually better at routine work than professional men. To correlate the material in a study containing hundreds of items, it is practically essential to make use of some method of machine tabulation.

The subject of medical statistics is extremely complicated, and much ground work is needed in the way of definitions and a tried morbidity list. The lack of these accounts to a considerable degree for the unsatisfactory nature of most administrative statistics and of those involving data from a number of institutions.

INDEX

Accident insurance, 14
Accident records, 46
Administrative staff, call for records, 55, 59
Administrative studies, 99
Admission
  data, 27, 36
  list, 66
American Association of Medical Record Librarians, 7
American College of Surgeons, 40, 100
  "Minimum Standard Requirements," 6
  hospitals rated annually by, 7
American Hospital Association, 7
American Medical Association, 7, 9
Anatomical plan of the *Nomenclature*, 73
  anatomical divisions, 74
Applications, data, 14
Arrangement of unit medical record, 33
Authorization and correspondence, 20
Autopsy
  report, 19
  permission to perform, 20

Bellevue Hospital, New York, 4
Binding, 32
Biopsy reports, 19

Card file, vertical steel, 63
Cards
  transfer, 55
  name, 62, *ill.*
  quality, 63
  combining clinic and hospital in one index, 64
  for diagnostic and treatment index, 67, *ill.*
  used in tabulating, 97
Case reports, first detailed, 2
Centralizing work of adding material to records, 32, 39
Check slip, 41
Chronological record, 12-22
  application data, 14
  initial examination, 15
  progress notes, 18
  special examination and treatment records, 18
  authorization and correspondence, 20
  clinic notes, 21
Circulation problems, 8
Clerical help
  hospitals asked to increase, 37
  better on routine work than professional men, 96
Clinic
  complicates problem of record, 34
  unified file contains records of, 47
  proximity of file to, 50, 59
  use of transfer card, 55
  records available to all members of hospital staff, 82
Clinic notes, 21, 42
Columbia-Presbyterian Medical Center, New York, 8
Compensation cases, 87, 89

INDEX

Complaint, 16
Condition on discharge, 29
Confidential information, safeguarded, 81
Consultation reports, 19
Content and form, 11-33
    front unit or index sheet, 12, *ill.*, 13
    chronological record, 12-22
    series of examinations and treatments, 22-25
    supplementary progress notes, 25-26
    summary sheets, 27-29
    format, 29-32
Continuation sheet, 29
    new, 39
Converting to reverse numerical filing, 50
Correspondence, 20
    with outside doctors, 88
Covers, 31
Criteria in a research study, 92
Cross indexing of names, 65

Damages, legal, interest of hospital in collecting, 80, 82
Definition and history, 1-10
    history of medical records, 2-9
Diagnosis
    provisional, 17
    final, conformity to nomenclature, 27, 41
    expected to conform to a certain nomenclature, 39, 41
Diagnostic and treatment index, 66-71
    card, *ill.*
    entry data, 67
    physical set-up, 68
    scheme, 69
    maintenance, 70
    section of, *ill.*, 76
    Standard Classified Nomenclature as basis for, 71-77
Diagnostic terms
    new, submitted to record committee, 43
    indexing, 70
Dictaphones, 38
Dictation, typing notes from, 37
Discharge, handling of record upon, 37
Discharge list, 66
Discussion groups, 7
Doctors
    approach of family doctor destroyed, 1
    significance of signatures, 29, 43
    assistance for, 37-40
    typing notes from dictation of, 37
    convenient place to work, 38
    adding miscellaneous material, 39
    indexing introductory letters from, before patients appear, 65
    responsibility for, and access to records, 43, 82
    tendency to transfer responsibility for records to hospitals, 83
    practice of withholding names of, 86
    responsibility that might be put upon a retired doctor, 87
Duplicate numbers, 35
    records for one patient, 36

Egyptian treatises on disease, 2
Etiological categories, 74
    of the Nomenclature, 71
    groups, symptoms, and operations, 75
    regrouped for diagnostic index, 75
Evening shift, to do filing and handle emergency calls, 59
Examinations and treatments
    single reports, 18
    specialists', 19
    series of, 22-25
    graphic chart, 22
    temperature chart, *ill.*, 23
    standing order sheet, 24
    special laboratory sheets, 24
    serial therapy records, 25

Family doctor, unity and continuity of approach destroyed, 1

INDEX

Family history, 16
Fastening sheets to cover, 32, 39
Files
   possible to unify out-patient and hospital files, 8
   space and housing, 50-53
   arrangement of active, 51
   storage space, 51
   to save adjusting follow block, 50
   advantage of uniform, 52
Filing and transportation, 8, 45-60
   reverse numerical system, 49
   requisition-filler system, 53-56
   filing schedule: daily return of active records: order of work, 58
Filing of name cards
   only experienced clerks should do, 65
   promptness in filing cards for new patients, 65
Filing schedule, 58-59
   daily return of active records: order of work, 58
Filing scheme, 45-51
   unified, 45
   accident records and others, 46
   unit numbering system, 46
   periodic transfers, 47
   changing to a unified file or to a unit numbering system, 48
Fillers, *see* Requisition-filler system
Final diagnosis, conformity to nomenclature, 27, 41
Financial reports, 99
Financial status of patient, 15
Floors, reinforced, 53
Folders, 31
Follow-up notes, 22
Format, 29-32
   plain white record form, or continuation sheet, 29
   special printed forms, 30
   means of distinguishing various kinds of notes, 30
   paper and ink, covers, 31
   binding or fastening, 32
Form for collecting research data
   preparing, 95
   insuring completion of forms, 96
Front unit or index sheet, 12, *ill.,* 13
Functions of the record
   rights, responsibilities, and safeguards, 79-89
   functions as an individual medical document, 79
   as basis for medical study and research: use for personal affairs of patient, 80
   position of parties concerned, 80-83
   patient, 80
   doctor: state, 82
   hospital, 83
   as source of public health studies, 83
   safeguards within the institution to assure availability, 83
   to preserve from those who have no right to see them, 84
   dealing with outsiders, 85-87
   to withhold nonpertinent data, 85
   responsibility for handling outside business, 86
   compensation and litigation cases, 87
   subpoenaed records, 87-89
   compensation cases, 89

Graphic chart, 22, *ill.,* 23
Graph-ruled record sheet, 25
Guides
   numbered, 52
   in diagnostic index, secondary etiological, for common or important diseases, 75

Handling, improvements in, 8
Hippocrates, first detailed case reports, 2
History, 1-10
Hospital insurance, 14
Hospitalization period, 36
   previous record, new admission data, 36
   new hospital sheets, 37
   discharge, 37

INDEX

Hospitalization summary, 27-29
 admission and discharge sheet, *ill.*, 28
Hospital record
 unit medical record the ideal form, 1
 idea of tapping for morbidity data, 8
 see also Unit medical record
Hospitals
 rated annually, 7
 safeguard against suits, 20
 many forced to maintain distinction between ward and private records, 79
 interest in collection of insurance or other claims, 80, 82
 position and responsibility of administration, 83
 safeguards within: availability of records at all times, 83
 chief danger, 84
 compensation and litigation cases a source of income to, 87
 subpoenaed records, 87-89
Housing of files, 50-53
 adequate space in convenient location, 50
 active records, 51
 records in storage, 51
 microphotography, 53
 reinforced floors, 53

Identification of the case, 14, 34-36
 unit record number, 34
Incomplete records
 current index, or file of, 41
 periodic reports on, 42
Index
 master name and master diagnostic, formed, 8
 unified in- and out-patient, name, 64
 diagnostic, 69
Indexing, 61-78
 name index, 61-66
 diagnostic and treatment index, 66-71

 standard nomenclature as basis for, 71-77
 symptoms: operations, 76
 secondary indexes: microphotography of old indexes, 77
Index of incomplete records, 41
Index sheet, 12, *ill.*, 13
Individual, the whole, as unit of medical practice and study, 1, 11
Initial examination, 15-18
Ink, use of colored, 31
Institution, safeguards within, 83
 see also Hospitals
Insurance
 accident or hospital recording of, 14
 interest of hospital in collection of, 80, 82
Insurance companies, hospital's proof-of-death form for furnishing data to, 86
International Cause of Death List, 4

Laboratory reports, 18
 adding them to records, 39
Laboratory sheets, 24
Legal evidence, state may demand record as, 82
Letters
 inclusion in record, 20
 doctors' introductory, 65
 to outside doctors, 88
Librarians, *see* Record librarians
Litigation
 complications of, render safeguarding of records difficult, 80
 temptation to misuse patient's history, 85
 cases a source of income to hospital, 87

Machine tabulation, 98
Maintenance of record standard, 34-44
 identifying the case, 34-36
 period of hospitalization, 36
 assistance for the doctor, 37-40

INDEX

maintaining the record standard, 40-43
Manifestations distinguished in *Nomenclature* from disease entities, 72
Massachusetts General Hospital, 4
Medical document, function of record as, 79
Medical ethics, 81
Medical information
furnishing outside doctor or another hospital with, 81
responsibility for giving out, 86
Medical practice and study, unit of, 1
see also Study and research
Medical records
history of, in general, 2-9
shelving of, 52
see also Unit medical record
Microphotography, 53, 77
"Minimum Standard Requirements" of the American College of Surgeons, 6
Miscellaneous material, addition of to record, 39
Morbidity data
idea of tapping hospital records for, 8
list; 100
Multiple tabulating code, 99

Name index, 61-66
name card, 62, *ill.*
physical set-up, 63
scheme, 64
maintenance, 65
doctors' introductory letters, 65
admission and discharge lists, 66
National Conference on Nomenclature of Disease, 9
New record sheets, passed on by record committee, 43
New York Hospital, 3
Night shift, 59
Nomenclature, uniform diagnostic, 4
purpose behind establishment of a representative standard, 8
diagnoses expected to conform to, 39, 41
as basis for indexing, 71-77
modification of classifications of, for indexing, 74
see also Standard Classified Nomenclature
Notes
means of distinguishing various kinds, 30
ways of handling doctors', 37
clinic, 42
Numbering system, see Serial numbering system; Unit numbering system
Numbers, identification by, 34
combination of names and, 35
doctor indicated by, 67
use of numerical code on diagnostic index card, 68
Nurses, practice of withholding names of, 86
Nurses notes, 25 f.

Obstetrical entries, 69
Operations
report of, 19
nomenclature of, 73
indexing, 76
Out-patient work
importance of speed in, 19
problem of notes, 21
see also Clinic
Outsiders
dealing with, 85-87
safeguards, 85
responsibility, 86
requesting statistical data, 100

Paper, 31
Parties concerned in records
position of, 80-83
patient, 80-81
doctor: state, 82
hospital administration, 83
Patient
the whole individual as unit of

Patient (*Continued*)
  medical practice and study, 1, 11
  incidental use of record for personal affairs of, 80
  position of the, 80
  right to privacy: limitation with regard to record, 81
  notarized authorization from, required before giving out information from records, 85
  information supplied for personal business of, 86
Pennsylvania Hospital, Philadelphia, 3
Personal history, 16
Physical examination, 16
Presbyterian Hospital, New York, 2, 5
Present illness, 16
Previous record upon hospitalization, 36
Printed forms, special, 30
Privacy, patient's right to, 81
Privileged communication, 81
Progress notes, 18
  supplementary, 25-26
  nurses', 25
  social service, 25, 26
Proof-of-death form for furnishing data to insurance companies, 86
Provisional diagnosis, 17
Public health agencies, interest in hospital records, 8
Public health studies, use of medical records as source of, 83

Qualifying factors in a research study, 92

Record bags, 56, *ill.,* 57
Record clerk, responsibility in giving out information, 84
Record committee, 43
Record librarians
  registry and training schools for, 7
  responsibility in keeping records up to standard, 40
  responsibility in handling outside business of hospital, 86
  responsibility in compensation and litigation cases, 87
Records, *see* Unit medical records
Reports
  on record deficiencies, 42
  laboratory, 18
  adding them to records, 39
  autopsy: biopsy: consultation: operation, 19
Requisition-filler system, 53-56
  requisition-filler, 53
  tabbed variation, 54
  return system, 54
  transfer cards, 55
Research, *see* Study and research
Return system, 54
Rights
  responsibilities, and safeguards, 79-89
  functions of the record, 79
  position of parties concerned, 80-83
  safe guards within the institution, 83
  dealing with outsiders, 85-87
  subpoenaed records, 87-89
Rubber stamps, 21, 31

Safeguards
  within the institution, to assure records' availability, 83
  to preserve from those who have no right to see them, 84
  in dealing with outsiders, 85-87
  responsibility, 86
  in compensation and litigation cases, 87
Sampling by record committee, to judge quality of records, 43
Serial numbering system, 46
Service analysis of records, 100
Sheet, large, used to collect and tabulate data, 97

INDEX

Signature of doctors, significance, 29, 43
Social service notes, 25, 26
Social workers, call for records, 55, 59
Sorting bin, 58
Source material, 90-102
  outlining the study, 90-96
  preparing the form, 95
  insuring completion of forms, 96
  tabulating, 97-99
  other types of studies, 99-101
Space and housing, *see* Housing
Special examination and treatment records, 18-20
Specialists' examinations and treatments, 19
Standard
  maintaining, 40-43
  lay responsibility, 40
  professional responsibility, 42
Standard Classified Nomenclature of Disease
  history, 8
  as basis for diagnostic and treatment index, 71-77
  basic plan, 71
  manifestations or symptoms distinguished from disease entities, 72
  operations, 73
  constructing index upon, 73
  anatomical plan, 73
  modification of classifications for indexing: anatomical divisions: etiological categories, 74
  etiological groups, symptoms, and operations: common or important specific diseases, 75
Standing order sheet, 24
Staples, wire, for fastening sheets to cover, 32, 39
State, interest of, in medical records, 82
Statistical data
  from diagnostic index, 66
  collecting it from records, 90-102
  outside requests for, 100

Statistical reports, 99
Statistical summaries, 29, 91
  sample sheet, *ill.*, 93-94
Stickers, laboratory reports written on, 19
Storage, 47
Storage space, 51
  housing records in storage, 51
Study and research
  concept of the record as a basis for, 80
  source material, 90-102
  outlining the study, 90-96
  purpose, survey of material, unit of the study, 91
  criterion, variants, qualifying factors, 92
  listing of items, 95
  administrative studies, 99
  service analysis of records: outside requests for statistical data, 100
Subpoenaed records, 87-89
  compensation cases, 89
Summary sheets, 27-29
  hospitalization summary, 27
  of hospitalization, 29
  statistical summaries, 29, 91
  sample statistical summary sheet, *ill.*, 93-94
Supplementary progress notes, 25-26
Surgeons, felt lack of continuity in records, 5
Surgery, movement to establish standard for, 6
Surgical summary for collecting statistical data, *ill.*, 93-94
Symptoms distinguished in *Nomenclature* from disease entities, 72
  indexing, 76

Tabulating source material, 97-99
  methods, 97
  form, 99
Telephone calls, 85
Temperature chart, *ill.*, 23
Therapy records, serial, 25
Transfer cards, 55

INDEX

Transfers, periodic, 47
Transportation of records, 56-58
   record bags, 56, *ill.*, 57
   trucks, 56
Treatment index, *see* Diagnostic and treatment index
Treatment records, 18-20
Treatments
   single reports, 18
   series of examinations and, 22-25
   important ones on hospital summary sheet, 27
Trucks, 56
Typing notes from dictation, 38

Unified file, *see* Filing scheme
Unit medical records
   definition and history, 1-10
   content and form, 11-33
   arrangement, 33
   maintenance, 34-44
   filing and transportation, 45-60
   indexing, 61-78
   rights, responsibilities, and safeguards, 79-89
   source material, 90-102
Unit numbering system, 34, 46
   changing to, 48
Unit of a research study, 91

Variants in a research study, 92

Ward records
   many hospitals distinguish between private records and, 79
   available to all members of hospital staff, 82
Weeding out, inactive records, 47
   alternative, 48
Work places, convenient, 38

Bei Fragen zur Produktsicherheit wenden Sie sich bitte an:
If you have any questions regarding product safety,
please contact:

Walter de Gruyter GmbH
Genthiner Straße 13
10785 Berlin
productsafety@degruyterbrill.com